SIMPLE STEPS TO FOOT PAIN RELIEF

Also by Katy Bowman

Diastasis Recti (Propriometrics Press, 2016)
Don't Just Sit There (Propriometrics Press, 2015)
Whole Body Barefoot (Propriometrics Press, 2015)
Move Your DNA (Propriometrics Press, 2014)
Alignment Matters (Propriometrics Press, 2013)
Every Woman's Guide to Foot Pain Relief (BenBella Books, 2011)

SIMPLE STEPS TO FOOT PAIN RELIEF

The New Science of Healthy Feet

KATY BOWMAN, MS

BenBella Books, Inc.
Dallas, Texas

BenBella

BenBella Books, Inc.
10300 N. Central Expy., #530
Dallas, TX 75231
Send feedback to feedback@benbellabooks.com

Printed in the United States of America
10 9 8 7 6 5 4 3 2 1

Library of Congress Cataloging-in-Publication Data is available upon request.
ISBN-13: 978-1-942952-82-4
e-ISBN: 978-1-942952-91-6

Editing by Erin Kelley
Copyediting by Lisa Miller &
    Karen Levy
Indexing by Amy Murphy Indexing
    & Editorial
Text design by Silver Feather Design

Text composition by PerfecType,
    Nashville, TN
Front cover design by Connie Gabbert
Full cover design by Sarah Dombrowsky
Printed by Lake Book Manufacturing

Illustrations by Carol Gravelle, Cecilia Ortiz (Ch. 6; figure adapted from Rossi)
Photography by Cecilia Ortiz, J. Jurgensen Photography, Brad Kazmerzak (Ch. 3)
Models: Breena Maggio, Tim Harris, Michael Kaffel

Distributed by Perseus Distribution
www.perseusdistribution.com

To place orders through Perseus Distribution:
Tel: (800) 343-4499
Fax: (800) 351-5073
E-mail: orderentry@perseusbooks.com

Special discounts for bulk sales (minimum of 25 copies) are available.
Please contact Aida Herrera at aida@benbellabooks.com.

CONTENTS

CHAPTER 1

How much do you know about your own anatomy? Did you know
that you should be able to lift each toe by itself? Can you? If not,
the basics of foot motion will be a fun ride!

CHAPTER 2

Any former ballerinas or soldiers out there walking around with
their feet turned out? Why do our gait patterns differ so greatly
from person to person, but tend to be the same within a family?
(Hint: it's not only your genes!)

CHAPTER 3

Sometimes foot pain is created much higher in your body than
you realize. The way you stand can load tissue in the wrong place,
causing it to wear out before its time. Do you wear your hips out in
front of you? That's a good place to start looking for likely culprits!

Even though bunions tend to run in a family, their appearance in your family tree has a lot more to do with the way you learned to move your body and the footwear you are choosing to wear, as opposed to flaws in your tissue. Find a solution here!

The parts of a shoe go beyond the latest style. By learning to identify four main characteristics, you can make smart choices when it comes to improving your outfit—and your foot health.

What is it about a shoe, really, that limits foot health? Turns out that the four main parts of a shoe each have particular qualities that can increase the development of common ailments like hammertoes, plantar fasciitis, bunions . . . just to name a few!

Are shoes limiting the feet? Are high heels really that bad? If a shoe were implicated in ailments of the foot, knee, or spine, wouldn't it be on the front of every newspaper? Well, the research *is* showing something, and it's time to start talking about it.

Everyone knows they are supposed to exercise, but few of us know what to do with the muscles in the foot . . . and there are *a lot* of them down there. This chapter offers a simple, easy-to-follow program that will help you restore function to the underused muscles in the feet, as well as increase circulation to the tight, overstressed tissue of the lower leg.

CHAPTER 9

Taking the Next (First) Step

Do healthy feet require a complete closet makeover? Am I going to be banned from cute or cool shoes forever? How do I fit more exercise into my busy day when I can barely handle what is currently on my plate? Find those answers here.

CHAPTER 10

Guidelines, Recommendations, and Frequently Asked Questions

What if I don't have foot pain, but want to prevent it? What if I want to optimize foot development in my friends and family? Does footwear matter during pregnancy, childhood, and my later years? Included here are guidelines on footwear for various ages and stages in life. Come find out what is best for your (or your family's) feet!

A NOTE ON THIS EDITION

An earlier version of this book was published in 2011 as *Every Woman's Guide to Foot Pain Relief: The New Science of Healthy Feet*. It's been translated worldwide and has helped resolve the foot pain of thousands upon thousands of . . . women.

My solutions to foot ailments are simple. Not always easy, but simple. Make slight shifts to your body posture when you're standing and walking to load your feet in a new way. Identify areas in your foot that aren't moving well. Do some corrective exercises, and figure out which aspects of a shoe are limiting the strength of your feet. These simple ideas have a profound impact on foot pain, and so it wasn't long before women relieved of their foot pain were begging me to write a men's guide to foot pain relief, so they could share it more easily with their male friends and family members.

The thing was, with a few exceptions, all of the information in that earlier version was just as applicable to men as to women. Men suffer from painful foot problems and related ailments too, and I didn't want them to miss out on what is really a human's approach to healthier feet, so I've created a new version of the book that can reach anyone who needs it.

I've also taken advantage of the new version to incorporate some of the research that's happening around minimalist shoes—it's been an exciting few years in the world of foot pain. The minimalist shoe "fad" has come and gone, leaving in its wake some die-hard converts to a minimally shod lifestyle, reaping all the amazing benefits of healthy feet—as well as some people with pretty serious foot injuries, injuries that occurred when people jumped too quickly into minimalist shoes without taking time to undo the damage a lifetime of shoes can bring. Many injuries might have been avoided had they considered some of the information and exercises contained in this book.

So this version is for *everyone* who walks around on two feet and wants to do so pain-free—it's for every man and woman who wants to make his or her feet healthier and stronger, step by simple step.

FOREWORD

As a medical specialist of the foot and ankle, I have encountered complaints from patients suffering with a variety of problems, including corns, hammertoes, bunions, and heel pain. Any podiatrist would tell you that treatments for these conditions include orthotics, injections, padding, medications, and/or changes in shoes.

Patients have also visited me seeking a second opinion after they have been directed to undergo a surgical procedure. The explanation usually given to the patient is that the musculoskeletal problem has become a fixed structural deformity that cannot be corrected.

In spite of the many advances in surgical treatment, we must be aware that these are biomechanical problems, and as such are inherently more dynamic than they may first appear. Realize that the majority of these problems are not congenital, that we have acquired them from a lack of knowledge regarding movement, bad habits, and, many times, poor shoe selection.

In this primer on healthy foot mechanics, Katy Bowman amuses as she informs us about the many things we can do to keep our feet feeling great. She offers simple solutions that you can take advantage of and practice on your own. I have seen positive results among my patients who perform these exercises.

Ms. Bowman's approach to clinical biomechanics is novel, and it is revolutionary. Her insight into the complex area that is the foot is literally the foundation for total body wellness.

At a time of so much uncertainty regarding the future of health care, and the increasing prevalence of diseases like diabetes and obesity, you can take control of your own health by educating yourself about how your body works.

Simple Steps to Foot Pain Relief is a testament to the effectiveness of a specific exercise protocol to correct lower-leg ailments that are mechanical in nature. Empower yourself with this handbook; some relief may be immediate, and lasting relief may require diligence.

If Ms. Bowman is part of a revolution in how we approach our health, then the new paradigm will support only those interested in taking full responsibility for their own well-being. As the book demonstrates, wellness is out there for those who are willing to work for it.

Theresa Perales, DPM
Ventura, California

INTRODUCTION

There are many milestones along the path to well-maintained feet, and an increasingly common detour is the path to the doctor's office, pharmacy, or even the operating room to fix an ailment from the ankle down. Far from being neatly confined to your shoes, foot problems actually speak volumes about the future status of your knees and hips, ability to walk for exercise, and ultimately the ability to live your golden years as a mobile and independent person. The foot is involved in virtually every non-sitting activity we do. If we want to stay upright and active—and feel great at the same time—we need to know more about our feet.

Often people will tell me, "I am too old to make any significant improvements in my health," or, "My feet have been like this for so long, they will never change!" Both of these statements are untrue! The state of your feet right now is simply the reflection of everything you have done up until this moment. Human tissues are dynamic and adapt to the forces that are placed upon them. When these forces change, the tissues change to reflect the different habit. This is true whether it's a good habit or a bad one!

This book is about how you can fix your own feet. Although human body issues often seem complex—especially to those with little or no anatomical, physiological, or therapeutic training—solutions can be much simpler than they appear. Though not on purpose, this "healing is complex" attitude is frequently reinforced by the entire health care system. As pharmaceutical and technological sciences advance, it makes sense that these advanced treatments would be the first used. After all, the more advanced the treatment, the better it is, right?

In actuality, most ailments do not require expensive treatments, complicated products, or even pharmaceutical intervention. Most musculoskeletal issues—that is, ailments of the bones, ligaments, tendons, and muscles—are usually created by one very simple, easily evaluated, habit: *how you move.*

The relationship between *how you move* and *how your body feels* becomes more and more clear the better one understands *how things work* in the body. Inconveniently, the human body wasn't created with an easy-to-use manual for quick troubleshooting when a problem arises. But all hope is not lost. By working backward, any person with the right training in physics and geometry can figure out which joint positions create the most degeneration, which footwear choices can increase pressure on which tissues, and which patterns of gait, or walking, can reduce muscle strength and nerve conduction.

The science of *how humans move* is called kinesiology. Within kinesiology there are many subfields, including one known as biomechanics. Biomechanics is the study of Newtonian physics (things like gravity, pressure, and friction) applied to living tissues. My personal area of study is the biomechanics of disease and injury, and I am dedicated to teaching the basic principles of physical science to people just like you, for the purpose of preventing and reversing damage to the human body.

This book is also about something bigger than your feet (even if you have really big feet). This book will talk about ailments north of the ankles that are being influenced by the state of your feet—ailments created where other body parts are responding to the impact of your footwear. Because of the way our health care system is segmented, experts of the feet don't typically talk to the experts of the spine or experts of the nervous system. Medical experts are thoroughly trained in the biological sciences as opposed to the physical sciences; since we all look for solutions using what's in our own tool bag, those who research human ailments tend to look for solutions in chemistry (pharmaceuticals) or genetics.

From the biomechanical field, research on changes in human geometry and body positioning and how they create

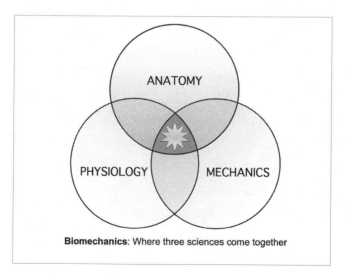

Biomechanics: Where three sciences come together

loading damage on tissue is only now emerging in the medical journals. The effects geometry has on physical forces like pressure, friction, and gravity, has been thoroughly understood in the physical sciences for hundreds of years. Geometry, along with the basic laws of Newtonian physics, applies as much to the human body as to any other physical structure in our universe. The more one understands the anatomical structures and physiological processes that drive human tissue regeneration, the clearer the picture becomes. This book will explain the mechanics of how common foot ailments develop in response to body geometry created by footwear and everyday postures. While the body adjustments may seem simple, keep in mind the science behind the solutions is as consistent as gravity itself.

Specific foot ailments vary, but in general, a foot ailment of any kind interferes with the ability of the entire body to function. There is hardly a human movement that does not involve the feet. No matter the current condition of your feet, you will find some piece of information in this book that will improve *how you move*, and in turn, improve *how you feel*.

A word of caution: this book is not a substitute for professional care but rather a manual on how things work in your feet, and how to alter habits that may be contributing to your problem. Human tissue is phenomenal stuff. When you make small changes in your movement patterns, you nudge yourself down a new physiological path. The body works to tear down old or underused tissue every day, and builds up tissues that are in greatest demand. The body continuously adapts to whatever you are doing *now*.

Changing your habits will change your life!

CHAPTER 1

Welcome to . . .
Your Foot

"He shifted his weight from foot to foot, but it was equally uncomfortable on each."

—Douglas Adams

First, let me congratulate you. Picking up this book is the first step toward improving the health of your feet, knees, hips, pelvis, spine, and bones. Most of what you are about to read was gathered during different parts of the academic research I did for my master's thesis. Using a force plate to see how shifts in hip position change the loads on the foot, measuring how flip-flops change your gait pattern, or observing how upper body curvature affects balance are everyday occurrences in a biomechanics lab. It is from these experiences that I designed the exercise protocol in this book, not only to make the foot healthy but also to optimize how the foot works with other tissues in the body. Through my corrective exercises and alignment suggestions—via books, DVDs, at our training center, or online—thousands have been successful in repairing their own feet by learning to change how they move. Some have shared their stories in this book to help motivate and inspire you and to illustrate that the solution really can be simple.

There are three likely reasons this book has called out to you:

1. You have feet.
2. You love the human body, preventive medicine, and anything to do with health.
3. As you are reading this, you have an aching, stabbing, soreness, swelling, stiffening, bunioning, smashing, cramping, and/or a limping sensation in your feet. You also have a closet of shoes, along with a vague notion that the two may be related. (Here's a hint: you're right.)

You have had your feet since birth. You've had them in your mouth, you've had them stepped on, and you have definitely had them squished into what seemed like a good style choice at the time. But chances are that you have no idea of the inner workings of your foot and ankles.

While you have about 200 bones in your entire body, 25 percent of them reside from the ankles down. The same goes for your muscles—a quarter of all the muscles and motor nerves in your body are dedicated to your feet. Despite all of these movable parts, I'll bet you've never been told this part of your body needs movement to keep healthy.

A keen student of the natural sciences, Leonardo da Vinci referred to the foot as the most complex piece of machinery ever designed. Don't let this statement mislead you, however, into thinking that understanding your anatomy is over your head. While the function of the foot is fantastically detailed, you will be amazed at how easy it is to navigate your way around a complicated area when you have a map. Wait, did you not get your map to the foot? Well, here it is.

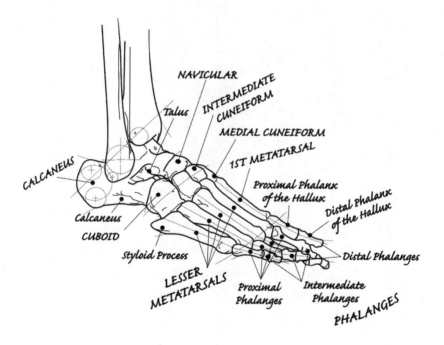

Okay, you probably don't need to know this much anatomy in order to successfully steer yourself to healthier feet.

That being said, you probably need to know a little bit more than this:

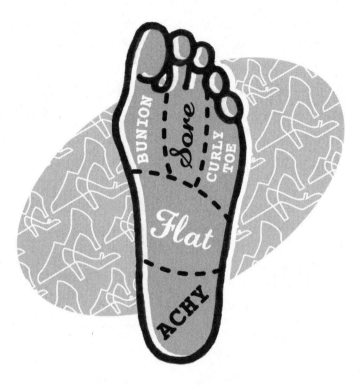

When it comes down to it, most of us know more about our cars than our bodies. Knowing the basics of automobile maintenance and performance parameters can significantly reduce the wear and tear on your car; the same goes for your anatomical parts.

To make significant headway toward healthy feet, you don't have to know the name of every single bone, muscle, tendon, and ligament that you can find in your feet, but you should know the general landscape and some basic terms.

In addition, a little information goes a long way when it comes to your ability to self-assess your ranges of motion, giving you an objective measure for your level of foot health. Knowing the correct anatomical terms will also help you to communicate with more self-empowerment, should you need to make a medical appointment. As a five-year-old, I'd have to point to a body location when the doctor asked, "Where does it hurt?" It's kind of embarrassing when you have to do the same thing as a thirty-, forty-, or sixty-year-old. With the number of baby boomers on the rise, and the steadily declining state of health across the country, the time has come to take more responsibility for our own personal health. Of course, if you are reading this book, you have already assumed that responsibility. Good for you!

THE HISTORY OF FEET

Feet and humans go back a long way. In fact, they go back all the way, right to the beginning. They grew up together, and evolved together, for hundreds of thousands of years before any shoes showed up on the scene. In the modern world, shoes have served to protect our living tissue from the unnatural surfaces that generate excessive forces, both at the surface (skin), and below it (bone). The increase of human-made debris has also created safety issues while walking barefoot through natural environments. Stemming from pre-antibiotic days when foot puncture could be catastrophic even for even a healthy person, footwear gradually evolved from light surface protection to completely engineered full-body stabilizers like

the hiking boot. Recently a whole new category of footwear—
"healthy shoes"—has emerged, along with myriad enticing
claims about how a particular shoe design can increase our
health or fitness levels if we do nothing more than wear them.

Footwear has evolved to a level of almost complete protection of the tissue from the environment. What began as the
protection of the foot has steadily become the encasing of the
foot, usually in materials more rigid than the feet themselves.
In other words, what da Vinci called "a masterpiece of engineering," a machine whose refined design evolved over mil-
lennia, is now stuck in one of your shoes. When an engineer
begins making repairs or modifications to any machine—
whether made of metal or organic tissue—the engineer has to
ask the question: What else might this change affect?

A biomechanist looking at the mechanics of the human
body will ask a similar question: For all of the benefit that
protective footwear may bring, what else might it affect?

Consider all of the bones and muscles that make up and
control your hands and fingers, and how many wonderfully
unique ways you can move them. The ability to type, play the
piano, conduct surgeries on microscopic tissue, and even but-
ton your shirt are all a result of learning how to use the muscles in your hands, and keeping them limber through regular
use. Now imagine that when you were two years old, someone
placed stiff, tight, leather mittens over your hands, lumping all
of the bones together, every day, from morning to night. Your
body would adapt to the situation, learning how to use the
muscles of the forearms and the joints of the wrist to a greater
extent. You would learn to use the outside edge of your hand

as one "finger" and train the digits to all work as a single body part. This way of using your hands would be completely normal to you, as that is the way it would always have been.

Now ponder this: the anatomy of your feet indicates the potential for them to be about as dexterous as your hands. However, the act of wearing modern footwear every day has created a mitten-hand situation in your feet—and you didn't even know it. We have weak, underdeveloped muscles within the foot and have placed large loads on the muscles of the lower leg, on the joints in the foot, and on passive tissues (those that cannot adapt strength) like the fascial systems and ligaments of the foot.

The good news is, by learning a bit more about your foot-machines, you can restore a lot of lost function and start the repair process right away. As long as your feet contain living tissue, they can change, grow, and improve, no matter what they've been doing (or not doing) up to this point.

Anatomy Lesson One: Your toes are separate structures from your feet for a reason.

When we think of the feet, we typically think of everything from the ankle down. Lumping this whole area together in our minds has the end result of lumping all the tissues together in our using patterns (or is it vice versa?). Each toe, just like each finger, has its own set of pulleys that allows it to function independently. While you'd be hard-pressed to come up with a modern activity that requires us to use our toes individually, using all of our parts serves a larger purpose. Every muscle has its own nerve supply that, when activated, keeps that local area of the body well nourished. While writing with our toes is not required for daily living (thank goodness—my penmanship is bad enough as it is!), being able to generate these movements is required to keep these parts of your body vital.

Anatomy Lesson Two: Your toes should be able to move separately from your feet.

Many people, especially those with chronic foot issues, cannot lift their toes without lifting their foot. Go ahead and try this. Stand up (it's okay, you can take the book with you), kick your shoes off, and see if you can lift just your toes without taking the entire foot with them. If you don't get it right away, try backing your hips up so your weight is over your heels, and keep practicing. You'll be surprised how quickly your toes may go from "zero" to "some movement" with a little practice.

Anatomy Lesson Three: Your toes should be able to move separately from each other.

Imagine all of the unique motions you can create with your fingers, lifting them one or two at a time, playing a piano, or even typing. We have the same potential in our feet as we do our hands, but we have casted these muscle groups via footwear, often for our entire lives, and so we have been left with stiff, weak, atrophied, and degenerating tissues in the feet. It's no wonder our feet hurt! If you had fun with the last exercise, you're going to love this one. Try lifting your toes individually, without bringing along the rest of the gang. I suggest starting with your big toe (see page 108 for an illustration of this motion).

Don't worry if you can't do it yet. You will learn eventually, with practice. In fact, many people who are without arms or hands train their feet to complete daily tasks—from diapering a baby, to writing, to playing the piano. We come with the necessary pulleys, levers, and electrical equipment needed for these movements—we're simply out of practice using them.

Anatomy Lesson Four: The front half of your foot should move separately from the back half.

Now that I've told you your toes are separate structures, keep in mind that the foot is not just one giant, fixed bone, but is made up of 26 bones and 33 joints. The primary reason our body even has joints is to allow for fluid movement. Could you imagine how hard it would be to use your arms or legs if your elbows or knees were missing? Your movements would be extremely rigid and stiff. The same goes for your foot: the less you use the many small joints within your foot by moving it in unique and novel ways, the less fluid control you have over stabilizing your body's weight—also known as balance.

Anatomy Lesson Five: There is no part in your foot that is shaped like an arch.

If you cut open the perfectly formed and healthiest foot, you would not be able to find an arch-like structure. Rather, the arch is a shape created by what the muscles and bones are doing. Wondering what happened to the arch of your foot? Think about arching your eyebrow. The work that goes in to lifting your eyebrow is similar to the muscular work that goes into drawing up the mid-foot. Only instead of using the muscles on your face, you'd need to use muscles in the foot, shin, and thigh. Said another way, if you want to restore the arch in your foot (or reduce an overly high arch in the foot), it's most helpful to think of the arch of the foot as an action, and not a part.

If you feel your high or low arches are giving you problems, you'll need to address both the strength and the flexibility of your feet. Whether your arches are completely missing, or high and stiff, the recommendation is the same: condition your feet with the Fit Feet exercises shown later in this book to develop strength and mobility in the right places for your body.

FOOT MUSCLES

Every muscle comes with its very own nerve supply. When you underuse muscles in the body, the communication between those nerves and muscles is less, resulting in a decrease in the health of both tissues. The inverse is also true: increasing the use of a muscle can improve the health of both that muscle and its nerve by increasing local circulation.

Increased circulation means more oxygen-rich blood (tissue "food") being delivered to an area and also a simultaneous removal of cellular waste products—waste that can otherwise accumulate and accelerate tissue breakdown.

The nerves that are responsible for moving the foot muscles originate from the lower parts of your spinal column. Traveling from your spine all the way to your feet, these nerves are some of the longest in your entire body.

The muscles of the feet can be placed into two groups: extrinsic and intrinsic. Extrinsic foot muscles are those with one end residing within the foot, and the other end residing somewhere outside of the foot. The muscles of your calves are examples of extrinsic foot muscles. Running between the feet and lower leg, these muscles move the foot around relative to the lower leg, but can't move the foot relative to itself.

Intrinsic muscles are those muscles that are contained completely within the foot. These muscles are much smaller, and are responsible for tiny, controlled movements of the many bones in the toes and feet. An example of an intrinsic foot muscle would be the abductor digiti minimi, the muscle that moves the little toe out and away from the rest of the foot. Ever heard of it? I didn't think so.

If we think back to the example of covering our hands with leather mittens, it would be the intrinsic muscles that would become underdeveloped due to lack of fine movements. It would be the extrinsic muscles working to compensate. In a chronically shod foot, the extrinsic muscles work more than they should and the intrinsic muscles work less than they should. Ideally, the work between the two should

ALL ABOUT YOUR PIGGIES

- In anatomical science, the toes are numbered outward, from the big toe (Toe #1) to the pinky toe (Toe #5).
- The bones in the toes are called foot phalanges (fa-LAN-gees).
- There are three phalanges in each toe except for the big toe, which has only two. This gives the smaller toes the ability to curl better than Toe #1.

be more balanced, with the intrinsic muscles functioning in coordination with the extrinsic muscles to walk deftly over natural ground, optimizing the shape of the foot arch and improving the nerve-muscle relationships of the foot.

FAST PHALANGE FACTS

TOE #1: *Hallux* is the Latin word for the big toe. It was derived from the Greek verb meaning "to spring" or "to leap." The big toe should be the last part of your body to leave the ground after your pelvis vaults into the next step, but often when the big toe joint is stiff, the entire foot must leave the

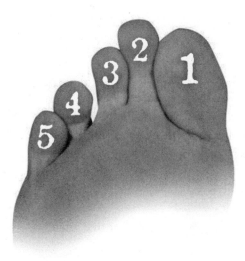

ground faster and as a single unit—and can result in a shorter stride length.

TOE #2: The second toe, also called the index or long toe, can be the same length or sometimes longer than the big toe. This condition is typically referred to as a Morton's toe. Oftentimes people will experience pain in this toe and be told that the longer toe is the problem. While a long second phalange will change the way the bones in the foot are loaded, damage to this area is caused not just by the toe itself, but also by a particular gait pattern coupled with the extra-long appendage. If you are dealing with pain and have a Morton's toe, you can change the mechanics of how you move to decrease the pain. Fun fact: the "Largest Morton's Toe" award goes to the Statue of Liberty.

TOE #3: Ask most Americans, and they'll tell you that this little piggy, the "middle toe," had roast beef. My Irish mother-in-law will say that this little piggy typically has bread and butter. How about we settle on a roast beef sandwich? Those with webbed toes (a not-that-uncommon condition called syndactyly) will usually experience the tightest bond between the second and third digit.

TOE #4: The fourth toe doesn't have a special name. Maybe that's why people wear toe rings, just to boost this toe's self esteem. This toe does have a greater risk for brachymetatarsia ("brachy"—short; "metatarsals"—bones in the foot), a bone that stops growing at a young age. Many people with a shortened fourth toe may notice some of the surrounding toes moving underneath, leading to painful walking patterns and "rubbing injuries" like corns and calluses.

Even though I have all my toes, I have been walking on only four toes ever since I was little. My next-to-pinky toe stopped growing at a certain age in my childhood, and that shorter toe has made it hard to find shoes that fit. Shoes either had to have lots of space in the front because the short toe sticks up (the pinky toe has curled underneath that toe to support it), or go high enough that they don't rub that toe and make it sore. Can you imagine cramming that toe into heels and walking without it hurting? Not a good idea, of course, but I have done it anyway, since high school! Your exercises and Earth-brand's wide toe box has helped me so much be able to spread my toes now and the shoes don't rub the top of my toe next to my pinky toe and make it sore. No more sore and aching feet! I am forever grateful!

—Lanene W.

Toe #5: This little guy got the cutest name of all: pinky. Typically the smallest of the toes, this little guy, unable to defend itself against fashionable footwear, is often greatly displaced when wearing your favorite pair of shoes and develops a corn as a response to the extra pressure or friction from the tight fit.

CORNEUM, CORNS, AND CALLUSES, OH MY!

There are lots of visual signs you can learn to read that give you insight into how you use your body. Corns and calluses are actually very clear visual signals that your body is experiencing excessive pressure or friction.

Have you ever wondered what a corn is, or how it got its name?

The top layer of your skin is made of dead cells and is called the *Stratum corneum*. *Corneum* is derived from the Latin word for "horned," as this layer is the oldest and "hardest" of the five layers that make up the outer layer of your skin.

The normal physiological response to mechanical irritation (increased rubbing or squeezing) is to "beef up" the area, to protect irritated skin. This thickening process is called hyperkeratosis ("hyper"—excessive; "kerat"—from the word keratin, a family of structural proteins; "osis"—the process of).

A "corn" is the small, kernel-shaped result of hyperkeratosis, which is a result of how your foot is interacting with its environment (shoe or landscape). A callus is the same thing, only more flat and broad compared to a corn. Corns are most commonly found along the outside of the pinky toe, although they can form wherever skin is pushing into something foreign. Calluses are typically found on the sole of the foot, where pressure (i.e., where you carry your body weight over your foot) is the greatest.

An interesting note: calluses are actually areas of the skin that have better circulation than other areas. What makes a callus uncomfortable is the fact that it is only a small area of thicker skin. This small patch of "health" becomes like a rock in a shoe (or a pea under a mattress if you're royalty).

If we walked barefoot over natural terrain throughout our life, we would prompt a gradual adaptation in foot skin thickness over that time, giving us a stronger surface to handle walking barefoot. Said another way, our feet are sensitive to walking over ground because they've adapted to footwear (i.e., the skin on the weight-bearing surface of the foot is too thin).

Key Points, Chapter 1

1. The anatomy of our feet indicate their potential to move in much more complex ways than we actually use them.
2. Allowing the muscles of the foot to go unused or underused allows muscles to atrophy.
3. Many foot problems are a result of disuse, combined with overloading the underused tissue.
4. The muscles in your feet are the same as the muscles in the rest of the body; they respond and adapt to regular use and specific exercise.
5. Retraining the muscles in the feet can increase the regeneration of the tissues that make up the foot, which can decrease disease and increase the overall health of your feet.

CHAPTER 2

Where Do *Your* Feet Stand?

"People are crying up the rich and variegated plumage of the peacock, and he is himself blushing at the sight of his ugly feet."

—Sa'di

O nce you have the basics of the anatomy of both the foot and footwear, you can begin to get objective about your own body. Before we start poking and prodding and measuring and quantifying your tootsies, you will need to remove your shoes. And yes, the socks have to come off too. You can't tell what your feet are doing until you can see them—clearly.

Now that you know a little more about your anatomy, it's time to get scientific and do some data collection. I'm going to walk you step-by-step through parts of your foot that you didn't even know you had! I've even included images and tasks to help you evaluate what is happening below your ankles.

We often forget that how our feet look is simply a reflection of how we have been using them. Lumps and bumps, calluses and dry patches, bone spurs, inflamed nerves, and even fractures are simply the result of what we have done with our feet. Undoubtedly genetics are a contributing factor, as various bone lengths and certain skin qualities increase the risk for certain ailments. Most genetic factors, however, are not diseases in themselves. Genes are simply qualities of human tissue that, when combined with particular habits or environmental conditions, might result in chronic pain or injury. But while you can't do much about your genetics, you can indeed do your feet a great service by developing better movement habits to ensure their long-term health.

The good news is this: the current state of your feet is influenced by many habits that are easy to identify and modify. The two habits we have that most significantly impact the structure of the foot's tissues are the shoes we wear, and the way we move our body. Footwear, as you will continue to learn, is responsible for a host of problems that directly contribute to foot pain and tissue degeneration. You have total control over what is in your closet, so footwear is really the easiest thing to change. When it comes to walking, you'll have to start paying a little more attention to your body in order to make lasting changes, but the payoff is worth it.

If you are reading this book, you have probably been walking for longer than you can remember. Even though just about everyone walks some amount every day, few consider how they actually do it. They just do it. Yet your gait pattern affects your body similarly to the way wheel alignment affects your car. And your feet are the best indication of where your foot "wheels" are pointing—and how many miles they have left!

NOBODY WALKS EXACTLY LIKE YOU

Your particular gait pattern (which is a fancy way of saying the way you walk) is an extremely complex, whole-body coordination system that is completely unique to you. Walking patterns are very similar to talking patterns. In the same way that the speaking accent you have is similar to that of your parents, the first influence on your "walking accent" was the way others around you moved. Like all animals, humans learn a lot about movement through observation. This is also why so many of us end up walking in a manner similar to our parents. After the initial pattern is set, your walking style is further enhanced by other activities you have done with regularity. Ballet dancers tend to develop a "ballerina turnout" even after they've left dance class. Those with military training keep the "at attention" feet long after anyone is checking. Walking with chronic pain, or even limping along after an injury—especially after a stint on crutches—can leave a person with an altered pattern that goes unnoticed (and thus uncorrected). And finally, many add a bit of their own walking "flair." These are little postural adjustments of choice.

We mimic the style of people we admire, or demonstrate an attitude or emotion we'd like to convey via body language.

All of these factors influence the position of our joints (including our foot joints!) and eventually, our alignment becomes a habit.

Your gait pattern can be measured and quantified with a lot of expensive and highly sophisticated biomechanical equipment. But here's a secret: you can also just look down to see what your feet are doing. This is a low-tech evaluation for sure, but still a highly effective way to see how you are moving. One interesting biomechanical tidbit about your body is that the position you have learned to acquire in order to balance while walking is the same alignment you maintain while standing. Analyzing your stance is easier when you're first starting—trying to walk and analyze your gait can be challenging.

WHAT SHOULD YOUR FOOT BE DOING?

As your body moves through each stride, many things are happening at the same time. The foot, in particular, should have four distinct positions it passes through while walking over flat ground. These positions are:

1. Heel strike—only the heel is planted on the floor.
2. Foot flat—the front of the foot comes down to join the heel and now the entire foot is on the ground.
3. Heel off—the heel leaves, but the front of the foot remains.
4. Toe off—the straggling forefoot and toes finally leave the ground and move toward another step.

In order for the foot to achieve each of these four specific points, the lower leg, foot, and toes have to be mobile enough to allow it. Tight calves, stiff ankles, and inflexible foot joints make this more difficult, and some of the points may be missed occasionally, or left out entirely! The "senior shuffle" is a walking pattern that bypasses most of these points, with the walker simply sliding a flat foot along the ground, or raising it minimally. Not only does a stiff lower leg and foot mean less muscle mass and less circulation, but it also increases the risk for tripping because it greatly reduces the clearance the foot has over rogue objects like cords and cracks in the sidewalk.

TAKE A LOOK

The best way to start off your foot analysis is to examine the position of your feet while standing in bare feet, in your normal, comfortable, everyday stance. I suggest you don't look at your feet until you have taken a lap around your room, looking straight ahead. Now stop, and settle into your comfortable stance without looking.

Now look down and take a moment to observe your stance.

First, check for symmetry. Are both feet doing exactly the same thing, or is one foot turned out more than the other?

Symmetry is just as important to maintain in the smaller segments of the body as it is when considering whole-body posture. As in any machine, working some parts harder than others results in different wear patterns. When it comes to

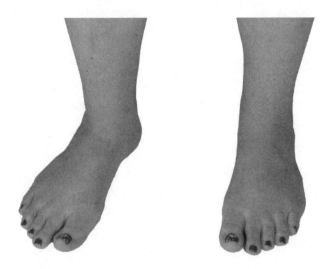

Would you drive a car with wheels aligned like this?

your feet, even wear of and between the feet is the key to strengthening underloaded areas and giving overloaded areas a break. A lack of well-distributed use can create skin patches that differ in resilience, bones that have spurs or less density than they should, and muscles that are used more or less frequently than what is optimal for the long-term function of the foot. The results of over- and underloading are typically considered to be ailments, but really, they are the tissue changes a biomechanist would expect to see based on use patterns. Your physiology isn't broken—it's working correctly! It's *the way* you're using your foot that's creating the problem.

The way you use your body on a daily basis changes its shape. We're a fairly sedentary culture compared to other human populations on the planet, and when we do move, it tends to be comprised of many asymmetrical activities, like driving, writing, or dominant-sided sports. Activities that use one side of the body more than the other affect how the musculature develops, and these muscle patterns, in turn, can pull on our bones in a way that reduces the overall effectiveness of our joints.

Symmetrical doesn't always mean that both sides of your body need to be positioned in exactly the same way. It means that the use of your body is fairly even over the course of a day or month, or even a year. For the corrective exercises in this book, you'll want

CONTINUED ON NEXT PAGE...

CONTINUED ...

to position yourself evenly, as the instructions will suggest, but keep in mind that the most balanced or symmetrical use of your feet doesn't only mean feet straight ahead all of the time, but that you are walking a lot, over different types of terrain, at different rates, on different surfaces. This is what truly challenges all of your foot parts and keeps most of your body used evenly!

There are other things that influence our general movement symmetry as well; an injury, for example, can cause us to shift our weight to the uninjured side to allow us to keep functioning while we're healing. All too often, however, a freshly healed person will fail to return to a more symmetrical pattern of movement. Or, perhaps when learning how to walk, you mimicked the nonsymmetrical pattern of someone in your household. No matter the reason, noticing the symmetry (or lack thereof) is the first step to reconciling your gait.

Second, check out the direction your feet point. Do they look like the wheels on a car, both pointing fairly straight ahead (better for the ankles and knees), or do they veer away from the center of your body (harder on the ankles and knees)? Maybe you've got one going forward and the other veering off.

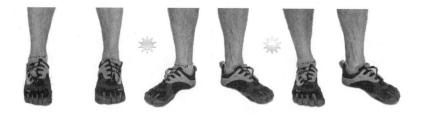

Your wheels point forward on the car because this is how a wheel propels your car straight forward. When wheel alignment is off, the motion of a misaligned tire against the road pulls the car forward and sideways at the same time (i.e., diagonally). As a driver, you can correct, or compensate for, the sideways pull by constantly turning the wheel in opposition, but this takes a toll on both you and the car; as you force the car to straighten out, the tire—and your arms!—wear prematurely. The same holds true for the non-forward-pointing foot. When the foot isn't positioned to push straight back, every step can push you to the right or left. In this case, the muscles in the back of the lower leg that should be propelling you forward are not able to do their job, and muscles that have other responsibilities are now required to compensate for them.

The greater the turn-out of your foot, the less your foot moves through the normal heel-toe cycle, and the more it lands on the outside of your foot, rolling in toward the inside of your foot. This disrupts the normal heel-toe cycle of forward propulsion, and replaces it with an outside-to-inside cycle. Or, more simply, you have a weight-bearing piece of machinery that is working in a direction it wasn't designed to handle over the long-term.

When we look at the direction a foot is headed, sometimes we are really only looking at the toes. The toes seem to be pointing straight ahead, so that must mean the foot is, too, right? Actually, when measuring foot position, it is best to look at the outside edge of the foot—not the toes or the curved instep. Using the straight edge of a carpet or yoga mat, check to see how far the outside portion of your foot deviates from the border. Try moving the outside edge of your foot until it lines up with the straight edge of the carpet. How does that feel? Odd? Odd is okay, and probably good for your foot.

TURN-OUT: A MATTER OF PERSPECTIVE

Many experts will argue that there is a *natural* turn-out to the foot, even though these data come from measuring the gait of modern, affluent, culturally sedentary, chronically shod populations. It is true that reviewing data in this way will show that almost everyone in our culture does, in fact, have a slight turn-out to the foot. But this does not prove that there is a *natural* turn-out to the foot—only that most of us have one after using our feet in a particular way.

If you consider the cultural habits most Western Europeans have shared for the last few hundred years, you will see two common trends: military training and ballet. Each of these traditions has a strong, enforced postural component. The "turned-out feet with heels together" posture is culturally inspired, as opposed to a natural foundation (meaning "from nature"). "Normal," "common," and "regular" are different from "natural," yet the many protocols that use dance as a platform tend to portray this turn-out as universally correct alignment, as opposed to alignment that is correct specifically in the context of dance.

We learn movement from our elders, teachers, and movement therapists, and nearly everyone is teaching turn-out, either explicitly or by example. Yet, when you actually examine the engineering of the toes, foot, joints, inner foot, and lower leg musculature, the position of the foot and ankle best suited for repetitive leverage (i.e., walking) is more straight ahead.

Even when data are collected in a scientific manner, it does not mean the conclusions are always valid. Think of the data collected for today's populations—weight, fitness level, hamstring flexibility, etc. Our physical states—even our skeletal positions—are still a direct result of user habit. It would be a shame if the textbooks of the future referenced the bone density or blood sugar statistics of today's population as "natural" just because that was the measures repeatedly found.

CONTINUED ON NEXT PAGE...

CONTINUED ...

After walking with an excessive turn-out for a long period of time, turning your dogs straight ahead will likely result in you feeling more turned in. That's because your feet are more turned in! You're not turned in too much (you can use the outside edge of the foot as a gauge), but probably a lot more than you were before. No, you don't have to turn your feet all the way forward while you walk; you can start by turning in a little, and then more and more as your lower legs become more supple through the correctives.

Once your feet are pointing forward, you might find your toes are curving in toward the midline of your body. That's okay, too. They've been like that for a while, you just probably never noticed. If you have been walking with your feet turned out for a long time, your toes may have realigned themselves to stay pointing ahead, even though the foot itself is turned out. As you strengthen the neglected muscles in the toes (see exercises on page 107–110), you can improve the muscular tone and impact their position as well.

Speaking of the toes, how do they look? You can check for symmetry in the individual bones, comparing those on the right foot to those on the left. Toes, even though they are pretty small pieces of machinery, possess the ability to do a whole lot of interesting movements. They can move to the right or left. They can lift up off of the floor, curl down into the sand, and they can twist and turn—especially if your gait is less than optimal.

Toes without well-developed musculature can get pushed around by the way you use your feet. In the same way a pitcher throws a baseball, your toes are being "thrown" by how you walk. For example, if you walk straight ahead with a lot of turn-out, your toe bones are being thrown straight ahead, which, over time, is what curves your toes in relative to your foot. Without well-developed muscles to keep them stable, toes can end up in each other's space, creating a traffic jam of sorts. When one toe gets pulled too far in one direction, it ends up, literally, on top of your other toes. The movement of toes is usually explained to be a problem with joint instability, but keep in mind, the first line of joint stability is the muscular system. Yes, your toes can become hypermobile, but that's usually due to not using your feet evenly and thus not keeping all of your foot muscles strong enough to hold each toe in its place.

This is also a good time to see if you have any hammertoes. These toes buckle up above the others, and can rub on the inside of your shoe, creating redness, soreness, or eventually a corn.

Become a Photo Detective

Our major walking and postural patterns were set very early on, as we learned to move by mimicking those around us. The moral of the story is this: the state of your physical body is the sum total of *how you have used it*. But you don't have to take my word for it—if you've got photos, you can be your own alignment detective!

Find the earliest photos of yourself that allow you to pay special attention to your feet. In those first-year baby photos, how do your feet look? Use both the symmetry and position-evaluating skills you have just acquired to create an alignment timeline. Here is an example from my personal collection:

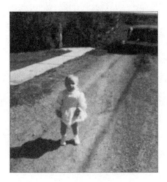

Here I am at about one year old. You can see my feet look pretty straight at this point.

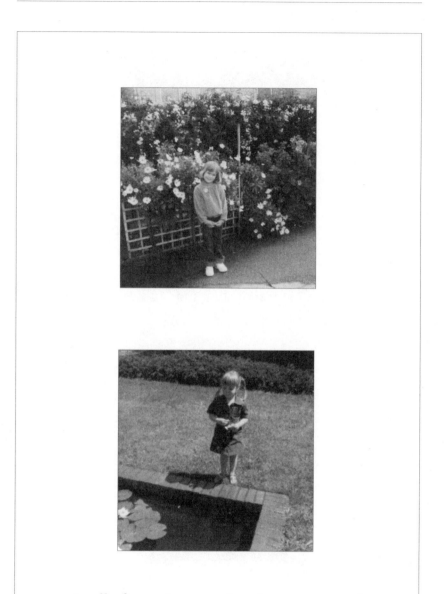

In all of my pictures taken between ages three and four, you can see that my right foot has started turning out.

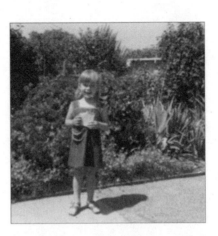

This is a pattern of standing (and walking) that stays with me for years.

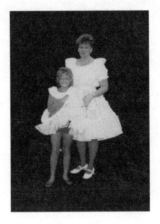

These pictures of my mom and me (who doesn't love a good petticoat picture?) show that someone else in the family has the same habit. Aha!

My detective work here is done!

Key Points, Chapter 2

1. Genetic factors certainly play a role in disease, but in many chronic conditions it is more *how* we use the genes we are given.
2. Two easily modifiable habits are the shoes we select and the way we walk.
3. Our pattern of walking is a result of observing how others walked while we learned to walk, in addition to dance, sport, or military training, and our personal "style."
4. Expensive equipment can evaluate our gait pattern, but we can just check it out in the mirror to make basic adjustments—for free!

CHAPTER 3

The Foot Bone *Is* Connected to the Hip Bone

"Toe bone connected to the foot bone
"Foot bone connected to the leg bone
"Leg bone connected to the knee bone . . . "

—"DEM BONES"

The direction your feet are pointing when you're walking matters, and there are other parts of the body that affect what is happening to your feet. Because the feet carry the weight of the body, every body part can affect the overall loading on your feet. Trying to figure out how every body part stacks over each foot can require lots of complex analysis, but there's one body part that's easy to measure that has a heavy influence on the health of your feet—your pelvis.

The pelvis relates to your foot heath because the pelvis houses your center of mass when you're upright, and wherever the pelvis sits over foot, that's where your foot feels the bulk of your weight. When people come to me with feet that hurt, the first thing I'll do is show them how to stand differently, so that they're not bearing down on that same place over and over again.

The densest structure of the foot is the heel bone, making it much better equipped for long-term weight-bearing than the small bones of the front of the feet. This isn't to say that your weight isn't shifting throughout the foot when you're moving, but when you're standing still, the musculature of your feet, butt, thighs, and core should be able to hold you fairly centered over the heels. (This is a good time to point out that keeping your weight over the heels is difficult, if not impossible, to do when you're standing in heeled shoes.)

FIND YOUR PELVIS

When you put your hands "on your hips," you are essentially placing them on the top of your pelvis, just above the actual hip joints. When standing, your pelvis should line up vertically with your knees and ankles (image on the left) as opposed to lining up with the front of your foot (image on the right).

When many people shoot for "good posture," they think "shoulders back," which often becomes "pelvis forward." Instead of shifting our shoulders back we're often just thrusting the pelvis forward. If you check out where your weight

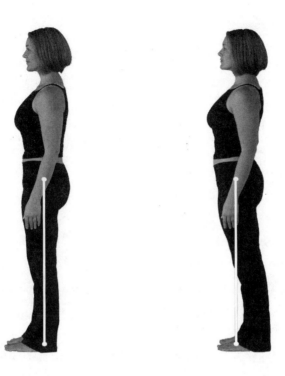

Vertical stacking,
weight over the heel

Forward pelvis, weight over the
front foot

falls in "pelvis forward," you might find that it's right over the achiest part of your foot.

When the burden is too great on the front of the feet, or feet squished into narrow shoes (more on that on page 69), the smaller muscles in the foot—muscles that *should* be focused on supporting the arch of the feet and dealing with the changing terrain underfoot—are overloaded with the constant weight of the body. Weight forward on the feet can also cause your toes to clench or grip (to avoid tumbling forward); the toe-scrunching motion is possibly a contributing factor to plantar fasciitis, hammertoes, and metatarsalgia (pain in

SPEAKING OF SKELETONS . . .

Everyone reading this book has either experienced bone loss firsthand, or knows someone who has been told of decreasing bone mineral density somewhere in their skeleton. Osteoporosis has become a national health care crisis as the affliction rate is not only increasing but also increasing in younger and younger populations. But where does it come from? The phenomenon of bone mineral loss has many components—nutrition, hormones, genes, and alignment. Wait, did I say alignment? Absolutely!

While your weight is fixed (in a moment), if you had a separate scale under your left and right feet, you could easily get the right scale to weigh more than the left by shifting your weight to the right. When we talk about "weight-bearing" in the body, we mean how much of your body weight is loaded onto it. When it comes to the weight-bearing status of your hip bones (an area prone to bone loss in our culture), where you wear your pelvis—out in front or back over your hips—matters.

Without a full understanding of the term "weight-bearing," many people are trying to increase the loading of their bones by adding hand weights or weighted vests to their daily walks and upping the resistance on the machines at the gym. These adjustments can absolutely increase how much you're working your body, but it doesn't always translate into an increase in weight-bearing status *of the hips*. And so, if you're really working hard toward healthy hips, then consider this: heeled footwear might not only be affecting your feet, it can also reduce the amount of weight you're bearing with your hips.

To better understand this, let us take a look at how bone regeneration works. When a bone is loaded (meaning the force of weight is put on it), it responds by maintaining a shape and strength (in the form of bone minerals) to support that weight. If you had tiny scales in each hip joint, the weight registering on these scales would go down as your pelvis moves forward. When you have a heel on your shoe, even a small one, the geometrical displacement of the entire body typically requires the pelvis to shift forward to compensate. And so, by having a positive heel underneath your heels with every step (and for practically our entire lives), we've decreased the weight placed on the bones of our hips, decreasing the signal to build bone in that area. It could very well be that, despite lots of exercise to build bone, the femoral neck, the part of the hip most sensitive to bone loss, is never directly targeted (i.e., can reap the benefit of your movements) simply because your footwear is preventing this area from receiving the osteogenic (bone-building) message.

the base of the toes). Stacking your weight over your knees, ankles, and the heels of your feet allows your body weight to be better supported by your skeleton, but most importantly, it instantly reduces the pressure on the front of the feet.

ALIGNMENT—THE QUICK FIX

Getting your weight back where it belongs is easy, fast, and free. I mentioned it before and I'll do so again: adjusting your weight off of your toes and back onto your heels is just about impossible when wearing a positive-heeled shoe. Shoes with *any* heel make a vertical alignment impossible because of the geometrical changes created at the ankle.

When barefoot, try backing your hips up, getting your weight far enough back to lift your toes off the ground. Your best friend in this endeavor? A plumb line. To create one, hang a washer on a string or use an exercise tube (be careful not to let the bottom touch the ground; it should be free to hang in line with gravity). Look in a mirror to see if you can get your hips, knees, and ankles lining up with your plumb line. You won't always have a plumb line with you, but if you try this a few times in the mirror with this objective measure, you can get a sense of how far back you need to move, and call on that feeling when you're out and about, standing in line at the store or bank.

Once you learn to evaluate posture using objective markers (like a vertical line), physical forces like loading and joint torque are easier to understand. Test your mechanical eye to see if you can identify which image features a "forward" pelvis. In other words, which picture below shows the front of the foot bearing more weight (i.e. the hips bearing less)? (The answer is at the end of this chapter.)

Backing your hips up until they make a vertical line with the knees and ankles might make you feel like you're sticking your butt out. First, get a more objective picture by looking in the mirror, as what you "feel" and what "is" can be two different things. While it's true you might be sticking your bum farther back than you're used to, it's not "out"; it's just back. Also, start paying attention to how your body feels when you're barefoot and stacked vertically compared to when

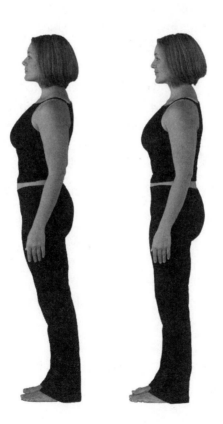

you're wearing a shoe with a heel. The more mindful you are about your body, the more you will start to feel different tissues squishing into position when you slip something onto your feet. You are being shaped by your shoes!

> *I was diagnosed with a bone spur on the top of my foot at the base of the big toe. It was very painful, red and swollen and limited my walking because it hurt all the time. I went to the podiatrist for his input and he told me the pain would "continue to intensify until a year from now I would be begging him to do surgery to correct it."*
>
> *I started making changes with my stance and walking pattern. The "feet straight ahead" was very helpful, as was putting the weight on my heels and changing all of my shoes to flats or negative heels. It wasn't long before my pain and the redness went away and with no swelling, I was able to enjoy walking again pain free. Well, I have continued to follow your alignment guidelines and still no pain after nine months! It even seems to be a bit smaller!*
> —DIANE L., PHYSICAL THERAPIST

(Answer: The picture showing more weight on the forefoot is the left picture!)

Key Points, Chapter 3

1. Pelvic position can play a role in chronic foot ailments, as its position can load the tissue in

the incorrect places, i.e., the front of the feet, as opposed to the denser areas of the rear foot.

2. Chronic pelvic placement can be a mindless habit—start paying attention to how you're wearing your hips.

3. It's almost impossible to get your pelvis off the front of your feet without getting out of positive-heeled shoes.

CHAPTER 4

Are Bunions Genetic?

"Even if genotype is the most important causal factor, in practice it is irrelevant, as it is impossible to modify one's inheritance but easy to improve footwear."

—I. B. SHINE, M.D.

I was recently watching a popular doctor-hosted daytime talk show when I heard the host inform his millions of viewers that bunions were genetic. I almost fell out of my chair.

More common in women but also occurring in men's feet, the bunion is often presented as an unpreventable condition, stored in your genetic code, just waiting to pop out and make walking painful and wearing shoes difficult. This is not the case.

Let's talk about bunions. The term bunion possibly comes from the Greek language, meaning "small hill, mound, or heap." Or, it may come from the Latin word *bunio*, meaning "enlargement"—who knows? The development of a bunion is usually a response to unnatural loading occurring along the joints of the *hallux*, which, as you'll remember, is the Latin word for the big toe.

As mentioned before, the toes on a foot can be displaced based on how you use your feet. How you move, how and where you walk, how often you walk, and what shoes you walk in (or don't) are all factors in what makes a bunion. Repeated (and sometimes tiny) twists in a walking pattern can weaken ligaments in the foot, displace bones, and change the environment within a joint; each of these changes the function and appearance of your foot.

WHAT IS A BUNION, EXACTLY?

A bunion is a prominence—an increase in tissue development or swelling along the medial border (the side closest to the midline of your body) of the big toe—called exostosis—and is a benign overgrowth of existing bone. This bony formation is separate (but related to) the position of the big toe relative to the foot. In anatomy-speak, when the big toe veers off toward the pinky toe, it's called *hallux valgus*. No one knows at this point whether the bony formation is due to the big toe's bone being forced toward the pinky toe due to narrow shoes, or the foot rotating around the big toe due to an overly pronated ankle, or a gait pattern that creates a hypermobile toe joint. What is know is that, after a while, the big toe can be pulled, or displaced, toward the pinky toe so much that it becomes almost perpendicular to the other toes. Not only do *hallux valgus* and a bunion reduce the function of the foot, but they can also make walking very uncomfortable.

The incidence of bunions is hard to quantify, but depending on what study you read, the rates range from 0.9 percent of total population, 28.4 percent of adults, and as high as 74 percent in elderly populations. While the numbers tend to vary based on how the data are collected, the common themes in the literature demonstrate that bunions happen most frequently in women and in older populations.

For those of you looking down at your bunions and recognizing the similarity with your parent's bunions, it is easy to think, "Ah yes, my bunions are indeed genetic." But there is one thing to consider about the data collected by researchers—the population being researched. In the case of current bunion research, the populations being evaluated in all of the studies are the chronically shod. Very little is known about the incidence of *hallux valgus* before people wore shoes. Doing research on "foot mechanics" has really become research on "foot mechanics of people who have always worn shoes," which is an altogether different animal if we're making statements about whether or not an ailment is genetic.

To get a much clearer picture of where bunions come from, it would be ideal to study a population of people who had never worn shoes. However, finding a population of historically unshod people on our modern planet is just about impossible.

Fortunately, there was quite a bit of data collection from various barefooted populations in the early 1900s, measuring foot and toe angles just as these cultures were starting to wear shoes. Although some of the techniques of measurement were likely rudimentary, the values produced from these studies tend to show that in shoeless populations, the incidence of bunions occurs more naturally in about 3 percent of the population—not a rate twenty times that.

Some people have conditions in which their collagen content is genetically proportioned differently than others. Genetics certainly plays a role in all musculoskeletal ailments, as things like the quality of your collagen and the length and shape of your bones are always at play when it comes to how the levers work in your body; however, genetics don't work in a vacuum. If you are thinking that you may be in this low percentage, then the collagen issue would be in all the joints, not just the big toe. You'd likely be experiencing hypermobility and joint instability in many of your joints, and in different tissue types. If you don't already have knowledge of a whole-body collagen problem, your bunions are most likely caused by habits you picked up along the way.

BUT EVERYONE IN MY FAMILY HAS BUNIONS!

Before there is a bunion, there can be the long-term displacement of the big toe (any teeny-tiny toe box wearers out there?), or there can be an incorrect loading of the joint first, causing tissue growth that pushes the big toe out of the way.

The too-tight toe box is a primary contributor to the sideways motion of the big toe, along with the elevated heel, which increases the load on the front of the foot. When your feet are all squished together, the muscles between the toes pulling them together get very tight. Begin with a daily stretch of all toes, giving extra attention to the big guy (see exercises in chapter 8). Placing your fingers between each of the toes will help restore muscle length and joint range of motion. If you have a pretty significant angle on the *hallux*, spend some time gently stretching and pulling the big toe away from the others.

FOOT POSITION

Now let us assume that you have never worn shoes that pinched your feet. In fact, let's say you've never worn shoes at all. Bunions are made in other ways, too.

As we discussed earlier, there is a large prevalence of turned-out feet. Just look around the next time you go out walking in any public place. And as described, this turn-out creates an increased amount of side-to-side motion of the foot instead of the normal front-to-back motion. The sideways use of the ankle has the weight of the body rolling not off the tip of the big toe, as in normal gait, but rolling over the side of the joint, which loads the big toe incorrectly. More simply said, when then foot is turned out, the "bunion area" of the joint presses into the ground with each step!

Remember, the side of the joint is the side. That sounds obvious, I know, but joints have a structure just as your house does, and both follow the same engineering principles. The walls don't have the same weight-bearing quality as the foundation. When you walkon the "walls" of your joints, instead of the foundation, your body has to call in reinforcement in the way of building up these walls, which results in bony protrusions or swelling that you see on your foot as the bunion develops.

What makes bunions seem genetic is the fact that one of your parents (probably your mom, given the higher prevalence of bunions among women) probably had them, as did her mom, and her mom's mom, which seems like too many moms for it not to be genetic. Keep in mind that out of all the things that are handed down from generation to generation, cultural input is right up there on the list with genetics. Genetic hand-me-downs—like collagen types and bone lengths and widths—can certainly affect your physical state, but so can non-genetic factors, such as walking patterns, shoe choices, and exercise habits. Our habits are sometimes hard to change, but they are much easier to alter than our DNA!

In addition to straightening your feet and backing up your hips when you're standing, there are two simple things you can do right now to begin to load your bunion differently.

First, stop wearing shoes with toe boxes that are too small for your feet. Too-narrow shoes push your toes together the entire time you're wearing them. If you want to mobilize the big toe, you need to give it space; it's as simple as that.

Second, pay attention to your foot position *while walking*. You don't have to become fanatical, but if you want to allow the tissue to recover from years of incorrect loading, you need to change your loading patterns. Sounds tough, but with a little mindfulness on your daily walk, you can improve the health of your feet while improving your fitness level.

Both the available evidence and the laws of physical science indicate that the majority of bunions are induced through footwear choices and gait. And so, you can see why I find it unhelpful for a medical professional to announce, without any disclaimer, that a potentially painful and debilitating foot issue is your genetic fate, The End. Changing the symptoms brought about by a bunion, changing the strength of your feet, and even changing the position of the bones within your foot are possible with corrective exercises and adjustments to your alignment and your footwear.

Key Points, Chapter 4

1. The heavily angled joint position of the big toe associated with bunions is called *hallux valgus*.

2. Research in shoe-wearing populations shows the incidence to be much higher in women and older-aged populations, and is believed to have a genetic component.

3. Research on non-shoe-wearing populations shows that the natural incidence of *hallux valgus* tends to be much lower than among shoe-wearing populations—only about 3 percent.

4. Long-term wearing of tight toe boxes can impact the soft tissue responsible for stabilizing the first joint.

5. Small habit modifications (simple exercise, correct-fitting footwear, and gait alterations) can instantly impact how you're loading your toe joints.

CHAPTER 5

Your Shoes . . . a Map

"I did not have three thousand pairs of shoes. I had one thousand and sixty."

—IMELDA MARCOS

You've made it through the human anatomy lessons and you now know more about your feet than many people on the planet. Learning the parts of the shoe will be a piece of cake! There are only four parts of the shoe that you really need to know. With this information, you will be able to improve your foot health and function by selecting shoes better suited to your feet.

I have briefly introduced the notion that wearing footwear is an unnatural habit that can reduce the function of your body. While I believe this to be accurate, it's also true that many of us have managed to compensate quite nicely as shoe-clad folks; we can walk, run, jump, compete athletically, and use our bodies quite well without really needing those smaller muscles. Until the day we begin to hurt.

With any bad habit, the damage we do to our feet accumulates over time, so we don't always see the connection between what we've done and how we feel. If you are a proactive health enthusiast, you should learn all about your shoes in order to prevent ailments from arising. If you are like most of us and are motivated by current pain, you will be able to figure out which shoe styles will allow you to increase your foot health and alleviate pain. Whether you are more motivated by prevention, pain relief, or both, you need to know how to evaluate your footwear.

If you are like many people, your shoes are likely purchased based on the activity for which you need them, such as sneakers for your exercise program, professional footwear for the office, or those going-out shoes that I like to call "killers"—the stiff and often heeled shoes (yes, men's too) you save for very formal occasions. Of course, that's just the starting point. If your footwear has fashion requirements, you might also have such considerations as the color (red), the material (patent), and how long you can walk in them (only until you find the next chair). You might already have your shoe shopping down to a science, with equations and three-dimensional graphs. Nothing against your current system, but be prepared to involve a new set of variables into your science. You need a new shoe anatomy.

Each part of the shoe has a unique way of changing the mechanics of the foot. Shoe designers, especially when it comes to athletics, performance, and "healthy" footwear, will often play with the geometry of each of these "parts" to get their shoes to do more than just decorate the feet.

Footwear design is very complex, with the engineer taking into account issues of pressure and joint instability. We're not going to get into all of the intricate parts of the shoe; all you really need to know in order to start increasing your foot health right away are the primary components that make up your shoe. Shoe anatomy is traditionally broken down into four main parts: upper, sole, toe box, and heel.

THE SOLE

The sole really is the "soul" of the shoe; it is for what footwear was originally intended. Designed to protect the skin from abrasions and punctures, what was originally a thin piece of animal hide has steadily progressed toward the impenetrable Fort Knox of Granny's orthopedic shoe.

The flooring of footwear ranges in terms of stiffness, thickness, squishiness, amount of contour (the lumps and bumps the manufacturer puts into the footbed), and height. Throughout recorded history, the soles of shoes have traveled the lines between healthy functionality and absurd heights, slopes and lengths, all in the name of fashion. Each of these characteristics can affect how your feet function relative to the ground, which impacts which muscles get used in the gait cycle.

THE UPPER

The upper of a shoe is the top-most material of the shoe and is what connects your foot to the sole. Uppers range from full coverage (like a sneaker), to forefoot-only coverage (like a mule or sandal without a slingback) to a flip-flop, or as I like to call it, the string bikini of footwear.

The qualities of an upper go beyond just the amount of material covering your skin; they include the type of material. For example, a water shoe has a stretchy, sock-like quality that helps your foot stay in the shoe, even if much of the upper itself has been cut away. Likewise, a well-engineered strappy sandal (and there are many of these on the market now) provides a good connection between the foot and the shoe *without* a lot of material. This means you can have a well-attached upper as well as the circulation of air over the skin of the foot, making this type of shoe ideal for warmer climates.

THE TOE BOX

There are two ways to measure a toe box. The first is its width. Take a long, hard look at the front of your naked feet and toes. All of that flesh and bone has to fit in the very front of your shoe, into what is called the toe box. Like all boxes, toe boxes come in a range of sizes—from the pointiest models of the stilettos you'll see on the red carpet to the wide, open front of a Roman sandal.

My first job in college was as a salesclerk at a department store. Women were required to wear skirts *(this was back in '95), so of course I bought my first pair of heels to wear on my first day—a "sensible" brown pair with a 2-inch heel. We were not allowed to sit down except during breaks, so my first eight-hour shift was excruciating! When I got home after work, I pried off my shoes and discovered that *both* of my pinky toenails were completely gone. I did not learn my lesson, though, and wore heels throughout college—and my pinky toenails didn't grow back until I got a desk job and found a nice pair of dress flats.*

—LINDA

You might think foot binding is a thing of the past, but when you consider some of the toe boxes that people today are choosing to squeeze their feet into, you might not be so sure.

The second way you can measure a toe box is how high it sits from the floor. Like the front of your bare foot, the toe box of a shoe should rest on the floor. At some point, shoe manufacturers started tipping the toe box upward, giving the front end of every shoe a sort of court-jester appearance. The next time you're in a shoe store, check out the fronts of all the shoes and see if all of the toes are flying just a bit above ground! (To see an image of an elevated toe box, go to page 135.)

ALL ABOUT YOUR HEEL

Finally, and perhaps most importantly, there is the heel. This could not be a book about foot health without giving all heel heights a little objective scrutiny.

The heel of a shoe aligns itself with the "heel" of the body. The heel is quickly becoming the most researched component of footwear, as this particular part has the ability to radically change the geometry of the human body. Just placing a little wedge under our foundation causes compensatory actions in the ankle, knee, hip, and spine, and can knock our natural gait pattern off-kilter—and it does this in an instant! The heeled shoe, believe it or not, has not always been just for women. In fact, some of the earliest versions of a high heel were worn by men, and still today, European and Latin shoe designers often use a lofty heel in men's dress shoes. The good old American cowboy boot sports a pretty hefty heel in its own right, which probably helps those cowboys reach their horses better.

Many people think they don't wear heels because they don't wear stilettos. Women are often trying to convince me that a heel doesn't really "count" if it's only an inch or two, and men and children's shoes don't come with a heel, right? Wrong.

> *I often wonder how many men have "bad backs" and traipse off to work in their heeled shoes—I have a swanky pair of men's dress shoes with heels that I like to wear to weddings. Which is ironic—the swanky part—since my back hurts so much by the time the reception starts that I take my shoes off for the dance floor before any of the women do.*
>
> —Michael C.

A heel is considered "positive" when it is at *any* height above the rest of the foot. So while we tend to categorize high-heeled shoes based on how they look, from a health perspective *any* shoe with a positive heel is going to affect the geometry of the body.

Replacing the term "high heel" with "positive heel" will help you figure out which of your shoes are affecting how you move. Once you start calling a spade a spade, you're going to notice that this new category of positive-heeled shoes includes not only traditional high heels but also the wedge, low pump, "business," and even running shoes. Who knew?

Key Points, Chapter 5

1. Footwear can be complicated, but simply knowing more about the four key design areas can significantly impact the health of your feet.
2. The four areas to evaluate are the sole, the upper, the toe box, and the heel.
3. Each of these areas has the potential to limit the natural range of motion of the foot and toes.
4. From an engineering perspective, the heel of a shoe is considered positive when it is any height above the toes, meaning if you were to remove all the positive-heeled footwear from your closet—you may not have any shoes left!

CHAPTER 6

Shoe Science

"Think of the magic of that foot, comparatively small, upon which your whole weight rests. It's a miracle, and the dance . . . is a celebration of that miracle. "

—MARTHA WASHINGTON

Here is something you already know: your footwear can absolutely affect the performance of your outfit. But here is something you might not have known: your footwear can absolutely affect the performance of your body. You may wonder why geometry is important when talking about health. You may have been told that you wouldn't ever need to do math again, but guess what? The long-term function of your body depends on how the particular bones, joints, and muscles are angled over time. Before going on to how footwear characteristics affect your body position, let's talk about why geometry matters.

MUSCLES—THE LONG AND THE SHORT OF IT

The muscles in your body, after receiving an electrical signal from your brain, change from long to short or short to long. These changes are called contractions, each resulting in a pull or release on the bones of the body, which result in both the movement you see with your eyes and the much smaller movements of fluids within the tissues. This smaller motion of fluid is called circulation, and the health of your entire body really depends on this process. Tissues that move frequently have better circulation than tissues that don't. The longer tissues go without circulation, the harder time they have continuing to grow (regenerate) and perform well.

So, back to geometry. Almost all of your muscles attach to bones. When you change the position of the bones, or limit the ability of the bones to arrange themselves into a particular configuration, you also affect the muscles that attach to those bones and the flow within and around them. The ability for a muscle to contract (which is how you get that circulation happening) depends on the distance over which a muscle can contract. The less range a muscle is given, the less it is able to change from one position to another (i.e., the less it can move) and the less circulation it can experience when moving.

Once you understand how skeletal position affects how the body works, it's easier to grasp why certain parts of your body—like your feet—aren't thriving. Shoes, and a lack of lots of walking over varied terrain, can, by proxy, "cast" your bones and muscles, limiting their performance and resulting in only localized delivery of nutrients. By restricting the distance and directions over which your foot bones can displace, you have minimized the activity of the foot muscles. This limit in foot muscle activity means limited circulation in the feet, circulation that is essential for the nerves, muscles, and skin of the feet and lower legs.

CIRCULATION—WHOSE JOB IS IT?

When we think of our blood circulating, we typically think of our heart as being the main driving force of blood throughout the body. In actuality, the same muscles that move your bones—your skeletal muscles—also play a significant role in distributing nutrient-rich blood throughout your body. The feet, being the farthest away from the heart, run the greatest risk of poor circulation; your cardiovascular system depends heavily on the movement of the muscles in the feet and lower legs

There are lots of factors that influence the movement of blood to the tissues, but if your feet have been locked up for a lifetime, training your foot muscles gives you a simple way that you can improve tissue health right now! See intrinsic foot strengtheners, page 107–110.

Shoes, in general, have characteristics that limit biological function, from reducing dynamic sensory input to limiting the ability for the foot to move relative to itself. There are four parts of a shoe, as described in chapter 5, that are the main culprits when it comes to affecting your whole-body geometry. By learning about them, you'll be able to find footwear that affords both protection and the mobility for improved strength and health.

THE SOLE

Before looking at what the sole of a shoe does, let us contemplate what the sole of a foot should be doing. In pre-footwear days, the sole of the foot sensed the natural surfaces we once walked over, forming itself with each step to meet and maneuver over these surfaces. It was this surface/sole interaction that kept each of the foot's 33 joints mobile, the numerous muscles supple, and the circulation pumping—resulting in very capable muscles, bones, and skin in the foot and the lower leg.

Just as your eyes and ears take in information about your environment, the skin is also a sense organ, taking in information about qualities of the surfaces it contacts. Exposing the skin to varying surfaces and temperatures creates a strong information highway between the feet and the brain, and the nerves conducting that highway are kept active and healthy.

As mentioned before, when shoes first appeared on the scene they were simple animal hides, tied to the feet with natural fibers. Their soles were thin enough to maintain foot mobility, but thick enough to minimize risk of foot puncture. When disease or infection from foot puncture places you at

NERVES OF THE FEET

There are two different types of nerves in the feet—motor nerves, which control the movement of the foot, and sensory nerves, which are responsible for "sensing" environmental factors like surface qualities (e.g., Am I stepping on something rough or smooth? Hot or cold?). Having both types of nerves working optimally means that, in addition to every muscle in your feet being able to respond to the movement commands coming from the brain (have you mastered lifting your toes individually yet?), your feet are simultaneously "reading" the environment. This environmental information helps the user of the feet (that's you!) make rapid adjustments with the motor nerves, selecting where and how to step to create safe passages for the feet.

great health risk, it makes sense to pick a shoe that offers the greatest amount of safety in the short term. However, as footwear has become thicker and worn for longer periods of time, we must also consider any harmful effects brought about by the long-term use of a shoe. If the same shoe you're wearing for protection limits foot sensitivity and mobility and, in turn, creates a deficiency in foot circulation, tissue health, and muscle strength, then you could very well have increased your risk of a foot ailment.

And, it's not only your feet wearing your shoes. When a part of the body is unable to perform its job, other parts of the body will compensate. In the case of foot musculature that is impaired or unused, the ankles, knees, and hips can develop compensatory movements, placing extra burden on these joints. The moral of this story: the thicker and stiffer the sole, the less the intrinsic foot musculature is able to do, the less communication happens between the brain and the feet, and the more compensatory movement at the ankle is increased.

THE UPPER

The upper portion of the shoe, when fitting correctly, would seem to limit foot function the least, right? After all, how much could a flimsy little flip-flop strap affect the gait pattern of a fully grown adult? Consider, for a moment, how a shoe stays on your foot. The upper is essentially a connection tool, designed to fasten the bottom of the shoe to your foot. As the upper gets smaller, so does the connection, saddling your foot with the responsibility of holding the shoe on.

Flip-flops, mules, and slide-on sandals are good examples of shoes that require a gripping action from the toes in order to keep the shoes from flying off while walking. This gripping motion of the toes is the same joint configuration and muscle tension pattern that deforms toe joints into the "hammertoe" position when done over and over again. If you don't believe me, try walking in your favorite pair of slip-ons with relaxed toes. It's fairly impossible, as your gripping reflex is so strong it happens automatically. If you have hammertoes, and you are wearing a shoe with a minimal upper, you are training your toes into the gripping motion with each step.

THE TOE BOX

The muscles of the toes tend to get away with doing very little over our modern lifetimes, as they have been squished into toe boxes since our first years. Throughout history, the square footprint has often been considered less attractive culturally, creating societal norms that include foot binding and the more subtle (but equally unnatural) tight toe boxes found throughout fashion today.

Just like a plaster cast limits the motion of a joint, typically resulting in muscle atrophy, the narrow toe space of most footwear prevents the spreading of the toes away from each other. Chronic toe squeezing not only weakens the muscles of the toes but also loads the bones while they are positioned incorrectly, increasing the occurrence of joint stress, bone stress, and other soft tissue deformation.

Because the square footprint was considered to be more "native" and therefore less desirable by the upper classes, the small-foot aesthetic is a sort of cultural by-product, handed down, often unknowingly, from generation to generation. Out of all the footwear characteristics, the squeezing of the toes into tight boxes has no suggested functional or safety purpose; it's simply a design component that has been elevated to the preferred look. A toe box that provides enough space for toe spreading and isn't elevated above the ground, forcing the toe joints into extension, allows the toes and their joints to load in their correct positions, decreasing unnecessary stress throughout the foot while standing or walking.

ABDUCTION AND ADDUCTION

The terms abduction and adduction are anatomical terms used to describe what a motion looks like. Abduction means "to move away from the midline." When the toes abduct, you can see them spread away from each other, creating space between the toes.

Adduction means the opposite. Just like "add" means to bring two numbers together, adduction means "to bring toward the midline." Adduction is the muscular action that brings the toes toward each other. Shoes (especially tight toe boxes) often keep the toes adducted. When your toes are adducted, there is no space between them.

Practice abducting and adducting your toes, trying to limit the curling or gripping action. Ideally, the toes should spread as easily as you can spread your fingers!

THE HEEL

There are a lot of parts to a shoe, but no footwear component is quite as geometry-altering—or as researched—as the positive heel. Why is everyone shocked that high heels are often linked to foot, knee, and back pain? Have you ever worn high heels? Have you ever *danced* in high heels?

When it comes to geometry, the positive heel creates an instant change in the angle between the foot and the shin that cannot be eliminated as long as the shoe is on the foot. Again, this stuff isn't rocket science; it's tenth-grade geometry.

We all start rationalizations for things we love at the same place: it's so small/infrequent/little, it can't really be creating this big/whole-body/complicated thing. I know, the small heel of a shoe hardly seems like enough to cause great problems, but keep in mind that although the height of a short heel may just be 1 or 2 inches, the foot is relatively short in length compared to the height of the body. Which means that the number of degrees that a 1- or 2-inch heel can displace the length (height) of you body is quite significant. What other machine do you know that you expect long-term use in positions that are 20, 30, or 40 degrees off their normal axis? Would you want to drive your car with the wheels 20 to 40 degrees out of alignment? What if your washing machine was perched at a 40-degree angle?

The higher the heel, the greater you've moved your body from a vertical stance (the first figure on the next page) to a compensating posture (the third figure). The middle figure demonstrates the amount of forward displacement created by

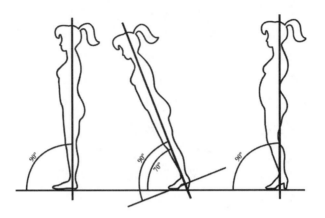

the heel (i.e., how much compensation is needed). People can compensate for the forward pitch with their ankles, knees, pelvic tilt, or spinal curvature. Any one (or all!) of these joints can be displaced to make the heel wearer look fairly upright, even if their bones are not truly vertical or loaded optimally.

The *way* a person compensates for their heel is based on many factors—their postural preferences and habits, the lengths of their body segments, their gait, and injury history. This is what makes it difficult to generalize the precise negative effects that a positive heel creates; each person copes with the displacement differently. But even if the compensations vary, the forward displacement created by the shoe is precise, and fairly easy to determine by a simple trigonometry calculation using heel height, shoe size, and body height.

In addition to whole-body displacement, the positive heel instantly increases the load on the front of the foot. If you're experiencing an issue of your toes or forefoot (front of the foot), then reducing your shoe's heel height can instantly decrease the loading that is increasing the pressure and furthering the issue.

"FIT SHOES"

A whole new category of shoes has recently come onto the market—"fit shoes." Distinct from athletic shoes, these are shoes whose makers claim, explicitly or implicitly, that you will become more fit simply by wearing them. Because these shoes have various features that are unique to their brands, they can affect your mechanics differently.

They've since fallen out of fashion, but when I wrote the first version of this book, the feature that fitness shoe designers were fiddling with most in order to affect the body was the curved (rockerbottom) sole, the theory being that if a surface is unstable, the body will have to use more muscle in order to stabilize itself. That absolutely makes sense from a physical training perspective. The result of using new muscle is usually an increase in overall fitness level, for as muscle mass develops so do things like total body lean mass and resting metabolism rate.

However, not all muscle development is good for the body's structural longevity. For example, I can clench my jaws tight all day long and—boom!—stronger clenching muscles. But what about the health of my temporal mandibular joint or my teeth as a result of my new jaw exercising habit? Although it seems logical to conclude that *any* muscle development is good, there is a way to use your muscles that's most beneficial for the health of the entire body. The arbitrary development of muscle, while perhaps contributing to over-all muscle mass, may have negative effects on the health of a joint or tendon.

The best way to evaluate your favorite fit shoe brand is to see how it holds up against our five-factor evaluation:

THE SOLE: Does the sole allow natural movement of the foot, or does it make the bulk of motion come from the ankle?

THE UPPER: Do I have to grip my toes to keep this shoe on, or does it connect well?

THE TOE BOX WIDTH: Can my toes spread comfortably, or does a too-narrow toe box reduce spreading space?

THE TOE BOX HEIGHT: Does the front of the shoe rest on the ground, or does it curl upward, forcing my toe bones into an extended position?

THE HEEL: Is the heel on this shoe affecting my other joints, or can I maintain a truly vertical alignment?

FAST FOOT MATH

For those math nerds out there, the foot presents a fascinating math problem just waiting to be solved. If I asked you how many unique positions you could achieve with your hands, it would seem to be an infinite amount—in fact, just playing one song on the piano would exercise your fingertips beyond their comfort zone.

There is a mathematical way, however, to solve problems like these. When trying to find out all of the possible ways your foot can be deformed, you can use an equation that raises the number of positions each joint can assume to the number of joints (33 in each foot). If we say, for example, that every joint can assume two positions (an underestimate; this is like saying your knee can only be fully extended or all the way bent), then the number of unique shapes your foot is capable of assuming would be 2^{33} (or 8,589,934,592) positions. And remember, this is an underestimate!

When we talk about things like human movement potential and really challenging our bodies, I like to keep these unbelievably high numbers in mind because they really demonstrate the potential of the nerves, bones, muscles, and connective tissues in our feet if we challenged them over a lifetime.

INSPECT YOUR FOOTWEAR

Aided by your new knowledge of footwear, you can now cast a more objective eye on the pair of shoes you wear the most often.

FIVE-FACTOR EVALUATION

If WEARING SHOES. . .	BEST	NOT TOO BAD		HARD ON THE BODY
Heel	Flat	Minimal positive, below 1/4"	Positive, 1–2"	Positive, more than 2"
Toe Box *Width*	Toes move freely	Toes have some space	Toes can't move	Toes are squished
Height	Flat	Slight lift before your foot is in	Elevated while standing	Elevated and stiff
Upper	Well attached	Sandal with heel strap	Slide	Flip-flop
Sole	Thin and flexible	Flexible, even if not so thin	Rigid, even if not so thick	Thick and rigid

A CHEAP WAY TO HEALTHIER SHOES

It can be overwhelming to contemplate replacing all your much-loved and perhaps expensive footwear with more foot-healthy alternatives. But there's another way you can begin to make changes to your shoe closet, especially in terms of heel height: power tools.

My husband has modified numerous pairs of shoes with a skill saw (yes, I can use power tools too, but most of the time I prefer to write books and he really likes to do things that make a lot of noise).

So far he has modified his work boots (he needed the steel toes, but not the heels) and soccer cleats (after he realized that it was the heel aggravating his back during soccer season; he's playing much better now, thanks for asking), some children's sandals that were perfect with the exception of the ¼-inch heel (why??), and a few pairs of sandals I've found through the years that just needed a little tweaking. Only once did we saw through, only to realize that the heel wasn't solid, exposing the inside of the shoe. Simple fix: We filled the holes with shoe-goo and they've gone on to be my favorite pair of boots.

In addition to sawing off the heels, you might find that some heels can be easily popped off if they've been simply glued or pinned on. If you're not feeling up to the task of 1) replacing your entire closet of shoes or 2) hauling out your tools and goggles, check with a local cobbler. Chances are you can transition your closet for a few bucks a pair!

DOES THE SHOE REALLY FIT?

Many people have spent their entire lives wearing shoes that are too small. Because we've been wearing them this way for so long, the sensation of tightly held feet seems quite normal. In fact, to many folks, shoes feel sloppy when they aren't pressing into the tissues of the feet. To get a sense of how much your shoes are affecting the way your foot can move, check how your shoes measure up against your feet, literally.

Try this: while standing, step onto a piece of paper without shoes or socks, and trace all around the outside of your foot (if you have a child to help you, they love this task!)

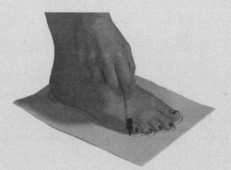

Step off and take a look at the size of your foot drawing. This is the shape your foot should be allowed to assume while under the load of your body weight.

Now, take out a few pairs of your favorite shoes and see how their size compares to the tracing. Many times, people will find their footwear is much narrower, especially at the toe box, than their foot actually is.

Key Points, Chapter 6

1. Muscle use plays a role in circulation, which is necessary to keep tissues healthy.
2. The amount your skeleton can move affects the amount a muscle can contract, which, in turn, affects the quantity of circulation coming through a particular area.
3. Footwear characteristics can instantly impact the position of your bones or the angle of your joints.
4. By knowing which footwear component affects each aspect of foot health, you can make better choices to improve your particular ailments.

CHAPTER 7

Undermining Our Own Health

"Sacrifice for beauty."

—My grandmother

As you've gathered from the back cover, this is the second edition of a book that was originally titled *Every Woman's Guide to Foot Pain Relief*. It always bothered me that the book was gendered—both men and women wear positive-heeled, stiff shoes, and we all suffer the consequences. I have deliberately de-gendered this edition because the information is applicable to pretty much anyone with a body. But there is no denying that all over the "civilized" world, women are suffering disproportionately from foot pain and related problems. Now that you have read the previous chapters, you can probably figure out why: their positive heels tend to be higher, their toe boxes narrower, and their pelvises farther out in front of them. Fashion has, via simple geometry, directly impacted the health of pretty much the entire Western world, and particularly women.

In an age of scientific research, one would assume that the reason this particular pitfall of women's health continues would be a lack of clinical data. But this is not so. There is enough research on footwear and inappropriate joint movements, excessive pressure, increased loading, increased risk of hip fractures, links to knee osteoarthritis, and alterations in pelvic placement and spinal curvature for someone in charge to say, "Your shoes, ma'am, might be making you sick."

It is easy to blame the current state of women's health on a historical lack of research, or a previous apathy toward women's issues in general. Feeling like a victim to our current physical pain or ailments is also an easy path. When taking a closer look at the link between our habits, our personal choices, and the constant struggle between what we know is the best thing to do health-wise, and what we tend to do, choosing poorly is an age-old habit.

Now granted, to a certain degree women may have already known this. Somewhere, a woman's good judgment must have had a reaction to a particular pair of shoes—you know, the ones she can't walk in for longer than an hour. Let's say that she only had an inkling in her subconscious. But let us say, now, that she knows better. She knows better, but she still wants to wear things that make her feel pretty and confident. I get it—totally. I've read Cinderella, too—Big Feet = Ugly Spinster Stepsisters. Ugly spinster stepsisters still living at home. To win the prince's heart, and live happily ever after, she must cram her foot into this tiny glass slipper. Seriously. Run that glass slipper through the five footwear evaluation points and you will find that while the upper passes the test and the toes are on the ground, the heel is too high, the toe box is big enough for only two toes, and the sole flexibility is zero. Good luck with that.

> *My first pair of high heels were the plastic ones they used to, and maybe still do, sell in the "girl" kits you'd find in the drugstore toy section. They often came with gaudy clip-on earrings, lip gloss, and such. I was about seven years old and wore them to bed the first couple of nights. That phase died out in me pretty quickly, thankfully, since I was one of the taller girls in school, not to mention a creature of comfort. Those darn things hurt! These days I prefer to be barefoot . . . which makes me truly feel like a little girl again.*
> —AMBER N.

Footwear can change the way we feel about ourselves. Shoes can make you feel taller if you're short, or authoritative when you need to feel powerful (ask King Louis XIV how he felt in his snazzy red heels). Shoes change the visual proportions of an outfit, distorting (subjectively improving) the way your body looks to others. And, the shoes in your closet always fit, even when the clothes don't. Shoes have become important to us because they make us feel better *psychologically*. And that's great, right up until they make us feel worse *physically*.

Early in 2010, a study came out about the harmful effects of heels and was covered on a national news show. The female anchor interviewing a doctor about what the study meant stated clearly, on national television, that it did not matter how bad they were for her, she would not be giving her heels up—ever. I encounter this attitude regularly. Despite the science, the research, the pain, and the visits to the doctor, some women find so much value in the psychological benefits of heels (feeling taller, thinner, more professional-looking according to this anchor) that they're willing to pay for that feeling with their health.

There have been other products in our culture that have provided the same psychological benefits—making us feel sexier, thinner, and more sophisticated—while simultaneously impacting our physiology in a negative way.

THE NO HIGH HEEL SECTION

I once came across a nutritional website asking if fast food would become the cigarettes of the future. I disagreed with the notion. There aren't many doctors across America who are going to be eating out of a greasy sack while you are sitting across the desk getting a prescription for high-blood pressure medication. I posted my own comment, hypothesizing that the positive-heeled shoe would eventually be found to be the main instigator in expensive ailments of not only the feet but of the knees, hips, and spine as well.

My comment was:

> I don't think fast food has become the "new smoking" as much as high heels have. Once upon a time, the

rationale for smoking was the sex appeal and the positive effect on weight management. Because it is hard to rationalize the choice of donuts as a positive one, poor food choices don't fit as smoothly into the analogy.

Bone-density-decreasing, nerve-damaging, and arthritis-causing high heels are probably being worn by your favorite OBGYN during your annual exam, eerily reminiscent of a 1950s doctor's visit, where Mr. Doctor chain smoked throughout your entire exam (anyone out there watch Mad Men?)

Blind to the detrimental effects footwear has on health, or the correlation of footwear to the gait alterations happening in the mother-to-be waiting in her office, the High-Heel-Wearing Women's Health Specialist doesn't know, in the exact same way Mr. Smoking MD didn't know, that when you look at the heeled shoe, you are looking at the "cigarettes" of the future.

I know, I know. Likening shoes to cigarettes is a pretty bold statement. And calling out doctors in heels as unconsciously promoting a poor health choice is also fairly bold. But think of this: a long, long time ago the cigarette, an item most would agree has a huge, negative impact on your health, was promoted by health care workers because there was no literature or research stating clearly that smoking was harmful to your health—until there was. And then there was a long time where people disagreed about what the research meant. And then it took a lot of time before people who smoked were able to stop, including people who truly understood the negative effects. Finally, smoking ended up on the list of clearly marked risk factors for many ailments, and insurance companies started taking note of who smoked and who didn't before giving people coverage. And if my prediction is right, so it will go with positive-heeled footwear.

INTRINSIC VERSUS EXTRINSIC MOTIVATORS

We have all decided to start a program at some point in time, whether for exercise or otherwise. What makes us successful at staying with these programs lies in what motivated us to start them.

Extrinsic motivating factors for exercise programs come from outside, like your doctor suggesting you begin a movement program for weight loss, or receiving a reward for completing a task.

Intrinsic motivation comes from the doer, as a result of the sheer pleasure or benefit one gets from the task.

Although you may have begun your foot health program in response to nagging pain (an extrinsic factor) or at someone else's suggestion, understanding the benefits, and feeling good after finishing each exercise can shift your motivation to intrinsic. Intrinsic motivation has been found to be an essential component of long-term success when it comes to physical improvement.

Until the research—research that already exists—begins to register on the radar screens of the people in charge of distributing health information to the public, there are things you can do to stop the perpetuation of the prevailing footwear paradigm of "keep your feet healthy by wearing stiff, supportive shoes with a heel." Just say "No!" to shoes that limit the performance of your body and "Yes!" to beautiful shoes that complement not only you and/or your outfit and/or your professional environment but also the long-term function of your human machine.

If you are a health care professional, understand that your footwear choices might be taken as inadvertent endorsements for healthy choices, and whether or not you feel it is your job description, you are a role model for health and wellness.

> *I have to admit, when I first learned about high heels and the damage they cause, I was sure I could "cut back" and wear flats more often. But after a year of learning more and more about alignment, and buying my first pair of negative heeled shoes, I find that now I hardly ever wear anything but flats. In fact, even my favorite cowboy boots, with their 2-inch heel, are gathering dust in my closet. Now that my feet don't hurt, and my toes are spread, there is no way I would stuff them all into a pointy-toed high heel. Plus, I feel more GROUNDED, better balanced, and am always ready for a long walk. THANK YOU for speaking out on this subject.*
>
> *—VICKI A.*

There is an abundance of research demonstrating the potentially harmful effects of footwear on the health of the human body. Even though the masses may not be dealing with this issue right now, you can be a study of one, and apply some of that data to your own body and see how your feet (and body) feel.

ADORNMENT

Before I had children, I assumed that the love of shoes came from the environment, but after raising some kids in a barefoot/ALL minimal-footwear household, there it was: one of my kids loved to stomp around in heels. We don't have these shoes in our house, as you can imagine, but it turns out access to "dessert" shoes is as rampant as access to sugary treats. Which is seemingly all. the. time.

It'd be a hard sell to say that a child has a natural affinity ("natural" meaning "as found in nature") for dressy shoes, but I'd totally buy that children and adults alike have a natural tendency to adorn their bodies, perhaps some more than others.

Comparing my two children (which is the most immediate sample I have), I have observed that my youngest prioritizes adornment more than my eldest. But in her habitat—of children's books and dress-up boxes at friend's houses—the only example of foot adornment seems to be smaller (plastic, pink, and sparkly) versions of high heels.

A few years ago, before I had children wearing shoes, I read an article on "Princess Feet." In the article, the author made the distinction between footwear and foot adornment. Once I recalled the article and this distinction, we went into full-scale "decorate your feet" mode—using paint, pens, stickers, and even mud to quench my kid's desire for adornment.

These were bits of holiday wrapping made into "flip-flops," proving that old adage that one person's trash is another person's flip-flops made out of trash.

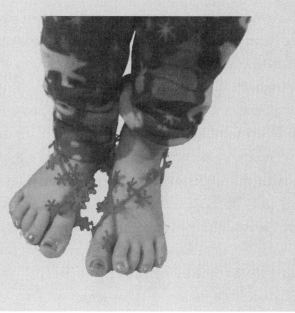

WHY IS REPAIRING YOUR FEET SUCH A BIG DEAL?

The function of the foot goes way beyond the scrunching of the toes and the stabilizing of the ankle. The foot is the platform for your entire body. The muscles in your feet need to be strong enough to keep your entire body moving as smoothly (and as long) as possible. If I haven't clearly stated it before, the current state of your feet is a future projection of how well you will be able to move as you get older.

When you're experiencing problems with your feet, consider that the issue is larger than the small area that's bothering you. You're a system, and the feet are but a part. Even though this book primarily addresses your feet, the health of your body depends on your feet. You may have never really thought about it before, but consider this: your ability to get up and get down, walk, and balance all call on the mobility and strength of the muscles within the foot.

Foot pain can also restrict the whole-body movements necessary to stabilize your blood sugar, preserve your bone density, and maintain your weight. Foot pain can prevent you from starting a necessary whole-body movement program. Walking, one of the most beneficial exercises you can do for your cardiovascular system, depends on the health of your feet! If your feet are too sore to go out, none of you gets to go.

You'd have to be living under a rock that's under a giant heap of dirt that's under another larger rock to have missed the fact that regular movement is key to health. Millions of people schlep themselves to the gym or yoga class, or head outside for a walk, to check off this daily to-do on the health list, and that's great. But what most people don't know is, they have unwittingly neglected the large portion of muscles that live below the ankle to a degree that might be infringing on future movement.

Often the most "fit" individuals—athletes, dancers, aerobics instructors, and marathon runners—have the least healthy feet. This painful truth is often blamed on overuse of the feet, instead of where it actually belongs—on the underuse of the foot. Or, more specifically, what happens when you regularly run, walk, jump, pound, and dance on top of weak feet.

Whatever your motivation is at this point—a reduction in foot pain, preventive medicine, interest in restoring alignment, or just plain curiosity—you are now armed with enough information to move into the exercise portion of this book, and toward stronger and more supple feet.

Key Points, Chapter 7

1. All of us, and perhaps especially women, often use footwear for "feel good" reasons, which can make footwear habits hard to give up.
2. High heels may someday be looked at the same way that we now look at cigarettes, which were also once highly fashionable.

3. There is an abundance of published research showing that footwear is a contributing factor to musculoskeletal ailments of the foot.

4. You do not have to wait for this information to become generally accepted knowledge before you can improve your situation—you can start using research findings now.

5. Foot health affects whole-body health; it's essential to begin your foot-health program as soon as you can!

CHAPTER 8

The Foot Gym

"The first step towards getting somewhere is to decide that you are not going to stay where you are."
—John Pierpont Morgan

No matter the state of your feet (or your shoe closet), you can absolutely make significant progress on your foot health via exercise intervention and habit modification. The great thing about human tissue is that it adapts easily, at any age. Really—it does. Before getting started with this exercise program, take a few moments to figure out with which level of foot training you should start.

Which statement best fits you?

STATEMENT ONE

1. I regularly go barefoot.
2. I wear high-heeled or highly structured shoes to work on a regular basis, but also wear flats or

flexible athletic shoes, or pad around my house in bare feet.

3. My feet are so sore, my doctor has recommended wearing shoes all the time.

Statement Two

1. I've never worn high heels or have, but only for a few dressy occasions.
2. I have four or five pairs of positive-heeled shoes (1 to 2 inches) in my closet that I wear regularly.
3. I wore high heels today to work. In fact, I'm wearing them right now, as I read this book curled up on the couch.

Statement Three

1. I jog or run regularly, usually four or five times per week.
2. I walk at least three times a week, and do some light stretching.
3. Balance has gotten more difficult for me. I don't feel comfortable standing on one foot without something to hold on to.

If you answered mostly 3s, it is likely that the tissues in your feet are extremely stiff. You will be starting with stretches of shorter duration and can use a chair or wall for extra balance as needed.

If you answered mostly 2s, you should be able to shoot for the mid-range of exercise time. You may find that doing the exercises more often, with a lower holding time, will be your best bet.

If you answered mostly 1s, then your feet, while still in need of specific strengthening, are probably up for the full recommended 60-second holds for each exercise. Some exercises may be more challenging than others, especially for athletes who have overused but undertrained their feet.

Because most of us have been wearing shoes since we were young children, we have missed out on learning the motions and exercising 25 percent of our muscles. The exercises in the "Foot Gym" affect the little muscles of the toes and those that support the arch of the foot, and also include the larger muscles down the back and sides of the thigh. These exercises are designed not only to undo years of accumulated weakness in the feet and ankles but also to help align the pelvis so your hip bones and pelvic floor can bear more weight and respond by strengthening.

PREPARING SPACE TO TRAIN YOUR FEET

To truly repair the foot, exercises for the feet need to be done without shoes. For those who have advanced neuropathy or diabetes, a concern is stepping on items that can puncture your foot without you feeling it. If you have very stiff feet, exercising on hard surfaces can also be challenging. To keep your feet safe, prepare a barefoot-friendly space before doing your exercises.

- Run a vacuum over your exercise space. A good vacuum will pick up smaller, hard-to-see items like sewing needles, pins, and tacks.
- Clear enough space to roll out a yoga mat or a large bath towel. This will give you an extra protective layer.
- For extra-sensitive feet, place your exercise mat on carpet, or layer a blanket or multiple towels to cushion your exercise space. (You can also do these exercises in socks if doing them barefoot is too extreme for you now.)
- Do a final, visual check for any potentially missed items.

These exercises require attention to detail. There are many things that change the effectiveness of an exercise, like the position of the feet, the bend in the knees, and the forward or backward lean of the torso. Learning where your entire body should be for each exercise will help you target the exact muscle fibers the exercises are designed for, and increase the overall effectiveness of the program.

EXERCISE ONE: Stretching the Calves

The muscles in the calves are significantly impacted by a positive heel, as they need to adjust immediately to accommodate, instantly, to any heel height. Long-term positive-heel wearing has been shown to shorten the fibers in the lower leg by 13 percent. Thirteen percent! (Check out Csapo, 2010 in the references to read more.)

There are many different versions of a calf stretch, and most of us have been given some type of stretch for this part of the body at some time or another, but not all calf stretches are created equal. This exercise is designed not only to load the muscles down the backs of the legs, but also to allow you to see how tension in your calves might be affecting your entire body while walking.

For this exercise, you will need:

- A full-size bathroom towel, folded and rolled
- A chair or a wall for balance

Start standing, facing the rolled towel.

Place the ball of one foot on the rolled towel, and gently lower that heel to the floor. Take a few seconds to straighten both legs all of the way, keeping the thigh muscles relaxed. Once you're used to this position, take a small step forward with the other leg.

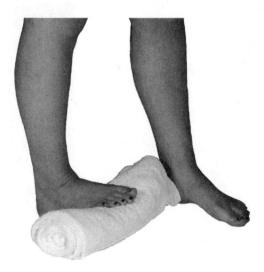

Ideally, your body should be stacked over your stretching leg. If your body starts leaning forward, or you have to bend either knee, scoot the foot on the floor back until you can maintain the stretch without these compensations happening. Use a wall or chair for balance if you feel wobbly. Step back and repeat on the other side.

Attention Pelvic Thrusters

Once you have taken a few passes at the calf stretch, start paying attention to the placement of the hips. The weight of the pelvis should stay directly over the stretching leg. Back your hips up until they stack vertically over the ankle and knee of the back leg. Maintain this hip position as you try to stretch your opposite foot farther forward.

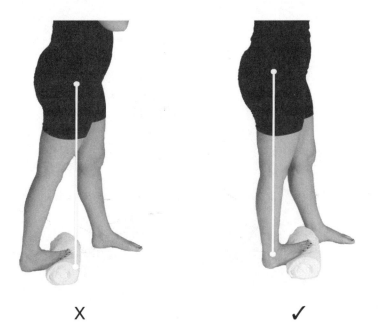

X   ✓

Other Postures to Watch

If your torso is leaning forward while stretching your legs, you have stepped too far forward. Shorten your "stride" until your body is stacked vertically. Only increase the distance between the feet if you can maintain your upright posture.

Helpful Tips: The thickness of the rolled towel makes this stretch more or less intense. If your ankle feels stiff, use a thinner towel, or don't roll it up all of the way. If stretching on this lower surface is still too intense, back the foot up just a bit to decrease the angle in the ankle. The same holds true for making the stretch more intense. For a greater stretch, choose a thicker or longer towel!

Why is this stretch so important?

Upright walking should be a smooth, controlled act that does little to damage the tissues. People, however, have developed a "falling instead of walking" habit that causes excessive loads on the joints and bones. The full range of the calf muscles should allow a step to happen without extreme pulling down the back of the leg, which shortens your stride in the long run.

The calf stretch is an easy way to measure how far you can step without being "jerked back" by the calf muscles. This stretch is also a great way to regain some of the muscle length reduced by any calf muscle adaptations to positive-heeled shoes. The longer you have worn heels, and the higher those heels are, the more challenging this stretch will be. Be patient and gentle with this stretch. If you have had a lifetime of muscle shortening in the lower leg, you can't undo it in thirty, sixty, or even ninety days. What you can do to increase the length is slowly wean yourself down to a lower heel and then to a flat, as well as pay attention to where your hips and torso are while walking around.

EXERCISE TWO: Stretching the "Gripping" Muscles

Although I am a fan of movement for health, not every exercise is beneficial for every person at each stage of his or her life. Instead, some exercises can actually worsen conditions because of the way they cause the muscles to shorten, and how that shortening affects the joints involved. "Towel scrunching" or "marble lifting" is a common foot-strengthening exercise often recommended to patients with weak or stiff feet, hoping that the increase in movement will help fix the issue. While this towel scrunching could possibly benefit someone with general foot or ankle weakness stemming from recent surgery, I am not a fan of this particular exercise as it's usually prescribed.

Just like the mechanics of wearing flip-flops, this toe-gripping action promotes a further shortening of the muscles in the toes that can lead to a decrease in joint range of motion. This "toe scrunching" motion is also the very same muscle pattern that can lead to hammertoes. If you're going to towel scrunch, make sure you focus just as much, if not more, on taking your toes in the other direction by unscrunching them.

Tight forefoot muscles stemming from overloading the front of the foot as a result of positive heels, excessive flip-flop wearing, or just years of poor posture, can generate tight, gripping toes.

This exercise not only stretches out the front of the ankle but also the toes if they have the gripping habit.

For this exercise you will need:

- A chair and/or wall to aid in balance

There are two ways to begin this exercise. If you are a 3 in terms of exercise readiness (see pages 93–94), then start seated. Those who are 1s and 2s can start standing, unless you prefer otherwise.

Reach one foot behind you, allowing the tops of the toes to touch the floor. If you are standing, you can start by reaching back from the knee, or, to make the stretch more challenging, you can reach the leg back at the hip. Try to keep both knees straight and your body upright. Be aware of your pelvis—it will tend to thrust forward to minimize the stretch!

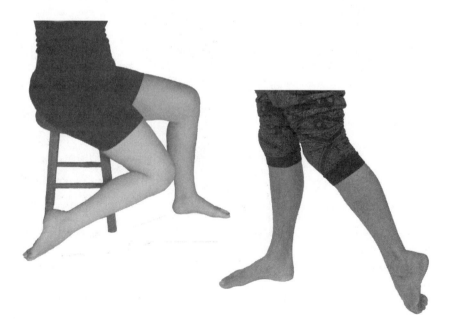

Attention to Detail

When the feet are very tight, the ankle will tend to roll out to the side (incorrect, image left), overloading the outer toes and avoiding the areas that most need the stretch. Bring the ankle back toward your midline (correct, image right), keeping the weight evenly distributed properly over the foot.

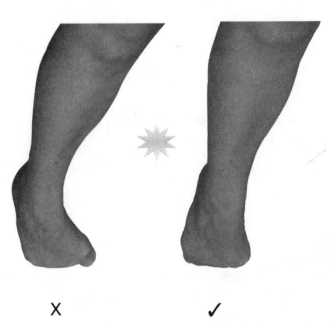

X   ✓

Note: cramping in the toes is very common while stretching them out after years of tensing them with every step. Feel free to start stretching in short bursts of time, seconds even, going back from foot to foot. You will notice the cramping subsides with regular practice.

When Will My "Grippers" Relax?

If getting your toes to unclench is your main priority, then take a look at your footwear of choice. If you regularly wear shoes with minimal uppers, shoes like flip-flops, poorly connecting sandals, mules, or clogs, your hammertoe muscles are working overtime to keep your shoes on. Make sure you're not undoing the effects of your exercise with your footwear choices!

If you have discovered you like to wear your pelvis out in front of you, or are fond of the positive heel, you might be causing the muscles to tense under the extra forefoot load. Reducing your heel height over time and minding your pelvis will help you keep your toe muscles relaxed and increase the long-term effectiveness of all of your foot exercises.

EXERCISE THREE: Lengthen the Backs of the Legs

When you have worn positive heels (and who hasn't worn positive-heeled shoes?) over a lifetime, the tension can affect not only the muscles in the lower leg but also the connective tissues running down the back of the thigh. Super-tight calf muscles can become super-tight hamstrings, especially if you have adapted to the geometrical changes of your shoes by slightly bending the knees. To move this stretch up a bit higher, we will add another piece of the puzzle.

For this exercise you will need:

- A chair
- A rolled towel

Start standing with straight feet, facing the seat of a chair. Bend forward, letting the hands settle flat against the seat of the chair. Back your pelvis up, until your hips are slightly behind your ankles. You may need to step a bit closer to the chair to do this easily.

If the backs of your legs are very tight, your muscles will pull your tailbone down to the floor. In this position, try to gently lift your tailbone up, away from the floor, increasing the stretch down the back of the leg.

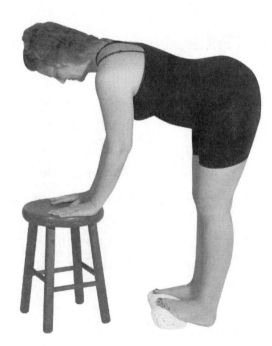

If your pelvis is extremely tucked in this exercise, stay at it with your feet flat on the ground. To increase the stretch, however, you can add the rolled towel under the front of the foot. Just like in the single-calf stretch, the height of the rolled towel affects the intensity of the stretch. For more stretch, increase the thickness of the towel; for less stretch, decrease the thickness, or remove the towel altogether.

Shoes Did All of This?

As a culture, we have not been very kind to our posterior leg muscles. Not only has chronic footwear use tightened the back of the legs but excessive sitting every day has also contributed to the shortening of these muscles. Stretching the backs of the legs can (and should) be done throughout the day, especially if you are a professional sitter. Keep a towel in a desk drawer at work for a quick leg lengthener three or four times a workday.

EXERCISE FOUR: Using the Wall

This is another, more relaxing way to stretch the back of the entire leg. Oftentimes, tight lower-leg muscles will cause the feet to point (plantarflex) while performing regular stretches. Using a wall prevents that movement from creeping in, and increases the effectiveness of your leg stretches.

For this exercise you will need:

- A pillow or sitting cushion
- A wall

Begin by sitting with your legs stretched out in front of you. Sitting up on a rolled towel, pillow, or multiple sitting cushions will help tight hamstrings and make this stretch a bit more comfortable. Scoot your body toward a wall, placing the soles of both feet flat against the wall. Pay special attention to your heels, making sure they are firmly pressed into the wall.

Relax your thighs. The knees should not be bent, nor should they be forced to the ground. If your legs are so tight

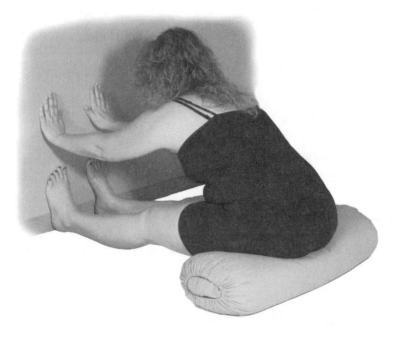

that they cannot straighten all of the way, increase the height of the pillows you are sitting on.

Slowly relax your body forward, trying to bend at the hips instead of the spine. If you can, reach your hands out to the wall. At this point, you can place your palms against the wall, or brush your fingertips against the wall, or gaze longingly at the wall, willing it toward you. Find the option that works best for your body. Finally, you can allow the neck to relax, letting the head drop forward. Take relaxing breaths and make sure you're not bouncing.

Why No Bouncing?

Bouncing while you stretch is called ballistic stretching. Often found in martial arts, the vigorous technique of a fast stretch and release has a place in sports where the body may need to prepare for the fast joint changes found in contact events. There's nothing wrong with bouncing, but it does mask the data you are trying to collect about your body, i.e., how far can you move with ease. Unless you are planning on competing in a full contact sport in the next few days, move slowly, and take some time to really become aware of how much tension there is in your body and how it's affecting your ability to move.

EXERCISES FIVE THROUGH TEN: Toe Lifts

Remember those small muscles within the foot, the intrinsic muscles? Just like your fingers move individually, so should your toes. Because the toe movement has been heavily restricted for perhaps all of your life, this exercise can take a while to master. In fact, toe lifts are actually five exercises rolled up into one!

For this exercise you will need:

- Your feet

Start with bare feet, pointing straight ahead. See if you can isolate the muscles that lift the big toe, getting it to lift off of the ground, without taking any of the other toes with it!

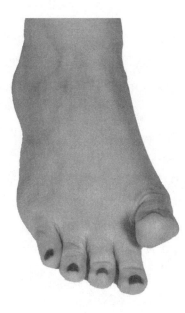

If this is easy, you can move on, following the big toe lift with a second, third, fourth, and finally, fifth toe.

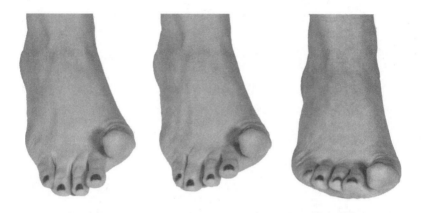

When lifting the toes individually, the foot and ankle should not change position, meaning you should not roll your ankle slightly to help you get the toes up. These muscles have muscles of their own, and these muscles need to learn to work.

If you are having a hard time getting started, you can lean forward to hold the other toes down to help your brain isolate the tissue you are trying to use.

Want Another Challenge?

After you have developed the ability to lift your toes up one at a time, you can also practice setting them back down in order.

Want Another, Even More Challenging Challenge?

Once you have mastered lifting and lowering your toes in order, you can practice lifting each toe off the ground by itself. This is much more challenging. Try picking up only your second toe. All of the other toes have to stay glued to the ground. Once you have figured out how to do that, you can start working on your third, fourth, and fifth toes. This one takes a long (long) time to master, so get to it!

Got Bunions?

If you have developed *hallux valgus* along the way, pay attention to the big toe as it lifts off the ground. Does it come straight up, or does it also veer off toward the pinky toe when lifting? In addition to your lifting muscles, you can take this opportunity to begin the arduous task of strengthening the big toe abductor (the muscle that stretches the big toe away from the others) while doing your lifts. Who knew doing foot exercises could make you break a mental sweat?

EXERCISE ELEVEN: Toe Spreading

Toes that have been crammed into tight toe boxes adapt to the limited space by squeezing together. This causes the muscles that pull the toes together (the adductors) to become tight and stiff, and the muscles that pull the toes away from each other (the abductors) to become atrophied from disuse.

A simple exercise to strengthen the toe-spreading muscles is to do just that; spread them! As often as you can, whether while barefoot or even when trapped in shoes, think toe spread!

For this exercise you will need:

- A foot
- A hand
- Something to sit on

Start by looking down at your parallel bare feet. Try to move the toes away from each other, creating space between each toe. Can you see the floor between them? As you try to get them to move away from each other, notice if they tend to lift up off of the floor or scrunch up in interesting patterns. This is all part of the process of learning a new movement program.

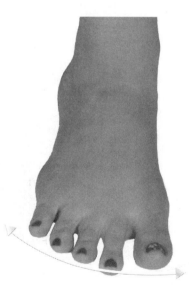

When you first start, the toes might not go very far. After all, it may have been thirty, forty, or even more than fifty years since you've played with your feet! To help them spread a bit more easily, try this stretch for the muscles in between the toes, or the toe's "inner thighs," as I like to call them.

Hold Hands with Your Feet

Sit in a comfortable position where you can get to your toes easily (crossing one leg over your knee works best). Place one fingertip between the tips of each toe, starting as far away from your foot as possible. Just placing your fingers in between your toes will give you a good stretch, but as these muscles begin to restore their length, you can work your fingers further down, until eventually, your fingers "hold hands" with your feet.

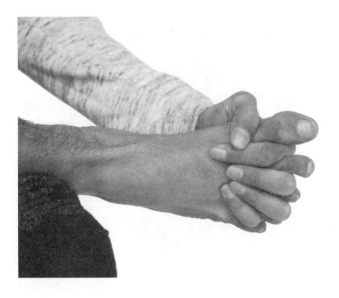

For more toe stretching, you can slightly spread your fingers, which will, in turn, move the toes away from each other even more. You can choose how much you want to stretch your feet. Give yourself plenty of time (weeks, months, years) to improve your foot health. After all, it took a long time to get your feet to their current state!

After taking your fingers out, try standing up and using your spreading muscles on their own. Are you able to spread better now?

Note: if you cannot get to your toes easily, you can ask someone for help. A massage therapist can help you with this stretch, or you can usually pay one of your kids a dollar (or twenty) to do it for you.

How Long Until My Toes Spread Easily?

Keep in mind that most shoes squish your toes together every minute that you wear them, so to undo hours of damage, hours of stretching are needed. Don't worry—I don't expect you to sit around with your fingers between your toes that entire time. There are a few inexpensive solutions that can work on your feet *for* you, while you are reading, watching television, or even sleeping.

If you've ever had a professional pedicure, you have probably had soft foam padding placed between your each of your toes. These "toe spacers" can be found at most beauty supply or drugstores and are usually less than $5. Pick up a pair and try popping them between your toes and let them stretch your toes while you sit back and relax. Or relax as much as you can, while your toes are being ripped away from each other. Just kidding. Stretching just feels like that sometimes, especially when certain tissues aren't used to moving.

One drawback to foam spacers is that they tend to stretch out after a few uses and are difficult to walk around or sleep in. Thankfully, there are new products on the market that are designed for this exact purpose. My favorite "spreading" inventions are toe-alignment socks and spacers created specifically to improve foot health. These items are designed for repeated, long-term use and can be worn while walking or in shoes.

> Our mother put us in sensible brown oxfords all through grade school and we hated her for it! When we reached the ripe old age of eleven, we were allowed to pick out and wear whatever shoe types we wanted. I was in love with a pair of light blue flats, which I bought in a size 7 1/2 even though my foot measured a size 8 1/2!!!!! I paid a dear price for trying to have my feet appear smaller! Years later, I have bunions, hammer toes, fallen arches, and one very bad arthritic knee!
>
> Thank you for introducing me to proper foot alignment and better shoes so that at sixty-four years of age, I'm finally able to spread my toes, have decreased the angle of my bunions and height of my hammer toes and can now walk for at least an hour with no knee pain!!!!
>
> —Chris D.

EXERCISE TWELVE: Get On the Ball

The foot comes with all parts necessary to walk long dis-
tances over natural surfaces. These surfaces were not only
bumpy and rocky paths but also yielding sands and firmly
packed dirt. Natural terrain also includes various and ran-
dom changes in surface. The contours of the earth kept our
feet supple by requiring them to form around many different objects. After wearing shoes for our entire lives, stepping
on objects feels excruciating—even smooth and broad stones
that couldn't really puncture our feet!

Because the foot is often held against a flat, unchanging
surface in the shoe, the numerous joints in the foot are not
encouraged to move individually. Stepping on surfaces that
vary in size and shape is what keep joints mobile, so to inner-
vate, or "wake up," these areas, you're going to get on the ball!

For largely immobile feet, a tennis ball or a ball designed
specifically for tissue mobilization (self-myofascial release
balls) is a safe way to introduce joint movement you have,
more than likely, never experienced.

For this exercise, you will need:

- A myofascial release/tennis ball

Start by placing just the front of the foot on the ball. Let
your foot drape gently over the ball. When you start working
with the ball, keep your heel down on the ground. Keep both
of your feet side by side and slowly move your foot forward,
an inch at a time, spending 20 to 30 seconds "just standing"
with the ball underneath that area. Once you have worked as

far back as you can without lifting your heel, switch to the other foot.

Once you have taken a "stance pass" with both feet, start again, with the ball underneath the front of the foot. After positioning the ball underneath your foot, roll your foot over the ball (keeping the heel down), exposing the sides of the feet to the sensation of the ball. You can progress on a time frame that suits you best. The more you explore the sole of the feet with a rounded surface, the more you will gently stretch muscle and move joints in a way that is completely unique and novel, while completely natural!

Helpful Tips: If your feet are very stiff, start working your feet on the ball while sitting down. Sitting reduces how much weight is over the ball, which reduces the pressure. Once you notice improvement, you can increase the pressure by standing!

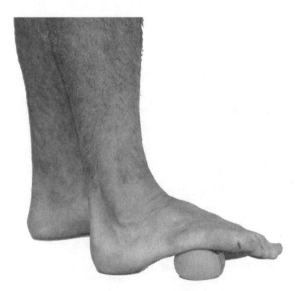

Attention Overachievers!

The ball is a great place to start, so take a while learning and benefitting from this exercise. If you are highly motivated to increase the range of motion in the 33 joints of the foot, you can take it to the next level. A few companies have come out with stone walking mats. Just like they sound, these mats have smooth stones glued or sewn to them, allowing you to practice walking on a cobbled surface without necessarily needing to bare it all outside. If you find walking on the stones to be too big of a step from a tennis ball, try laying out a bath towel (or two) over the stones to build up the smaller muscles in the feet. This will decrease the intensity of the surface, allowing you to adapt to it more slowly. Once your feet are stronger and more mobile, consider venturing out into your backyard to play with the movements brought about by the varying shapes and textures you can experience. To keep things safe, do a visual check for any items you want to avoid. You can also create a small "barefoot space" in your yard that's covered to keep out any harmful debris.

Key Points, Chapter 8

1. Create a safe "barefoot" environment before beginning your foot health program.
2. Try each of the exercises to see how you do on your first pass. Note which are easy and which are challenging.

3. Take your time on the exercises that are the most challenging, based on how they feel to your body.

4. Increasing the time spent on each exercise, and the number of times each exercise is repeated, or changing the angles of your body to make the stretches more challenging are all ways of increasing the intensity of the program.

CHAPTER 9

Taking the Next (First) Step

"You have brains in your head.
"You have feet in your shoes.
"You can steer yourself in any direction you choose."

— DR. SEUSS

As we approach the end of this book, you may be facing a quandary. You understand all the information I've given. You no longer desire to have foot pain (did you *ever* desire to have foot pain?), but perhaps you feel trapped, as many people do, between the desire for wellness and what seems like some big changes in habit. You have, after all, been wearing shoes, and possibly wearing high-impact shoes, for some time now. Below are some of the usual comments I hear floating around the hall after I lecture on the subject of the high-heel hangover. Do any of them resonate with you?

- I can't afford to replace my entire footwear wardrobe, nor alter all of my clothes, to accommodate a new, lower, heel height.
- I love my shoes and I feel [short; heavy; dumpy; less elegant; less professional] without them.
- I can't find the time to add an entire foot-training program into my day.
- It's so much easier to fix my problems with a shot or surgery.

And then there's the bit about walking. I know, you've been walking around your entire life in a particular way and now I am asking you to *change* how you go about getting from one place to the other? The nerve!

Believe it or not, I do not want you to feel overwhelmed. Feeling like there is a huge hurdle between you and health is only going to deter you from making the small (really!) changes that will give you relief. As a culture that likes to go big, we tend to attempt huge changes to our habits when we want to get better. When we want to lose weight, we go on ten-day juice fasts or eliminate all foods that start with "carb" from our diet. When we decide to start exercising, we go out and buy a three-year membership to a gym, a new pair of $200 running shoes, and five great workout outfits. What's the problem in these scenarios?

The change is too much and we are setting ourselves up to fail.

When we aren't eating well, the best solution for long-term success is to start by addressing a single thing, like soda. Or the fourth cup of coffee. If you're feeling ready to start exercising, what about adding a daily mile-long walk and take it from there? Want to feel less stressed? The solution is not, realistically, moving to India for a forty-day retreat at your favorite ashram, but rather fitting ten minutes of stillness into your day, with no cell phones, no talking, and no fidgeting.

An overzealous approach to health can cause us to crash and burn like a kid after a Halloween candy binge. So I'm asking you to look at starting foot care in a practical way. Actually, you have already made improvements to your health by simply reading this book. One of the biggest cycles we get ourselves into with chronic pain is feeling like we are a victim to it. Why is this happening? I am hoping you now have a better awareness about the foot and how issues are created, and are a bit more relaxed about where to go from here.

When you're ready, try out a few of the exercises. I don't recommend you start by doing them for thirty to forty minutes a day. This isn't a fitness manual, but a guide to testing the muscles in your feet. These corrective exercises don't require large amounts of physical effort. Each of the exercises can be done in one-minute increments throughout the day. I understand that finding a large gap in your schedule is challenging, so try running through a few of the exercises while brushing your teeth in the morning and evening.

Many of the guidelines given in this book can apply to things you are already doing. Paying attention to your gait pattern while out for your regular walk does not take any extra time, only a little extra attention. The same goes for adjusting your alignment while standing around in line at the bank or the grocery store. You can improve the health of your feet in seconds, simply by adjusting how you load them.

HOW OFTEN, AND FOR HOW LONG, DO I NEED TO DO THE EXERCISES?

At some point in our recent cultural history we developed a differentiation between exercise and movement. Exercise, by definition, requires a structured set of time, a level of intensity, a quantity of reps per session, and a number of sessions per week. The problem with thinking of alignment as a series of "exercise sessions" is that it implies that you don't have to think about where your body is in space all of the time, or at least, as often as possible. In order to change something as engrained as how you use your body, you have to think while you are using your body. And that means you have to think about your alignment often, going beyond the time you are doing the exercises.

Now that I have said that, there are general guidelines that will help you change your tissue sooner, rather than later:

- You should work up to holding each exercise for at least a minute. This might not be possible at first. You may find that your muscles cramp and protest, which is a fairly normal part of any exercise program. Use your body's reactions to the exercise as a guide for increasing or decreasing the intensity or the duration of each hold.

- The more frequently you do these exercises, the better results you will have. The minimum for each exercise should be at least once a day, but a good middle-of-the road habit to get into is cycling through the entire series of movements three times. Each time you run through the cycle, you will find the improvements to one set of muscles make it easier the second, and then third time. Use the exercise section at the end of this book for easy reference.

- Learn the gait alterations and the basics of each stretch, and integrate them into your lifestyle, permanently. You will more than likely be a shoe-wearer for the rest of your life, which means you will need to keep some sort of exercise program going for your feet for—well, forever! Keep in mind that the muscles in your feet are made of the same exact tissue as the muscles in the rest of your body. You don't think that the weight lifting you did ten years ago is still doing your body good, do you? The same muscle science applies to the feet, so keep up the good work!

WHEN WILL I FEEL BETTER?

The answer to this question is . . . it depends. The time it takes for your muscles to strengthen or restore in length depends on:

- What shape your feet are in now.
- The type of shoes you have worn throughout your life.
- The length of time you have been wearing shoes.
- Your particular gait pattern.
- How frequently you do your exercises as well as how frequently you move altogether.
- How frequently you think about and respond to where you carry your weight on your feet.
- The types of shoes, or the lack thereof, you choose moving forward.

For many ailments, the pain relief is immediate. If you have had the habit of bearing all of your weight on a particular area of your foot, to the point that you have developed an issue, just removing that weight can reduce pressure and change your situation in an instant.

Other ailments were created over years, or even decades. You can change your mechanics and make improvements on a cellular level that may not become apparent for years, although you likely will experience a gradual lessening of pain in the meantime. Whatever your experience is, know that whatever your original goal may have been (curing a chronic foot condition, for example), a new goal can be investing a small amount of time every day in ensuring healthier feet for the future.

When you start any exercise program, it is important to have small progress markers along the way. If you set a 20-pound weight loss as a goal, and lose only 12 pounds, would that make your program ineffective? Of course not. Apply that same mentality to the goals you set with your feet.

When coping with pain, it is common to see changes in frequency, intensity, and even location.

FREQUENCY: how often are you experiencing pain?

INTENSITY: on a scale of 1 to 10, is your pain changing, or is staying exactly the same?

LOCATION: is your pain in the same area, or does that area feel better but now you are feeling pain in new areas of your foot or lower leg?

Use these as markers to measure whether your new program or footwear is having an impact on your foot status.

MAKING OVER YOUR CLOSET

Whether you are considering changing 10 percent of your habits, or if you are excited enough to be thinking about changing out your entire closet, I have done my job well.

After reading through the suggestions and recommendations, you will find that it is not a requirement to toss out all of your footwear in order to get pain relief.

If you are ready to purchase footwear matching the guidelines appropriate to your feet (see chapter 5), I suggest getting a pair in which you will do the greatest amount of walking. Your habits of walking are where you'll find your most engrained movement patterns. You may be tempted to splurge on a pair of flat dress-up shoes that will be worn once or twice a week while sitting at your desk, instead of getting the flexible, negative-heeled walking shoe to use on your thrice-weekly, 2-mile walk. Choose the latter. Whatever shoe you will wear the most often while bearing the brunt of your weight is the best choice for your dollar. If you can get both, then get both. If you can get neither, then take a good look at your closet, find the lowest, most acceptable heel to you right now, with the widest toe box, of course, and make that shoe your staple. And, do your exercises every day.

> *I got my first pair of high heels at age thirteen and I thought I was just too cute, until an older guy laughed at me for being so wobbly. Devastated but determined, I practiced wearing them and finally succeeded—I even was able to run in them. I couldn't figure out why I kept getting backaches and finally herniated L5-S1 disc (duh). Went to chiropractic college to learn about the spine and learned about those wicked, but seductive, high heels. Bye-bye heels, although I too have a few pairs I hide in the closet that call to me in the night.*
>
> —GAYLE I., CHIROPRACTOR

I am often asked, "Do you ever wear heels? Ever?" Here's my answer from five years ago: I keep a pair of gold, strappy, heeled sandals in my closet. I bought them more than ten years ago and every time I spring clean, rearrange my closet, or move, I consider tossing them out. But I never do. These shoes make me feel like a Greek goddess when I imagine myself wearing them. I pick the outfit out in my mind, including the dress, the jewelry, and the hair. In my Greek fantasy, my hair is down to the floor in mermaid waves, just in case you were wondering.

All of this is true, actually. And so is this: I haven't actually worn these heels in five years. The first reason is, nowhere in my fantasy do the soles of my feet burn at the halfway point of the evening, or do I have to take off the shoes and put on a pair of scuffed backup shoes I found in the trunk of my car. Yet, both of these things usually happen whenever I wear heels.

Here is my answer today: I no longer have these, or any, heels, but thanks to the minimalist-type footwear that's come out, I have a much-loved pair of gold strappy flat sandals that please my inner mermaid and my actual biped.

I communicate with a lot (and I mean a lot) of people who can no longer walk without pain due to the state of their feet. Their inability to walk has translated into weight gain, or extended periods of time where an unfortunate sole (get it?) has battled depression due to constant pain with every step.

I have worked with seniors who are unable to maintain functional lives due to the fact that their stiff and painful feet have jeopardized their balance, to the point of being at risk for a fall simply by walking through their house. Many people I have seen consider hip and knee replacements, foot surgery, and cortisone injections as the norm.

Personally, I want more out of my physical experience than what stiff, heeled shoes can offer. I enjoy walking along the beach, using the power generated by my own muscles, for as long as possible. I like to hike long distance through nature, with my kids. I desire long-term function more than I want to live out my fashion fantasy that often comes with exorbitant price tags in the form of joint instability, chronic pain, and the reduced ability to move. The good thing is we all have that choice, and we can choose better, the more information we have.

My personal footwear choices are being barefoot often, using the very minimal shoes (i.e., strappy) for walking and hiking as often as I can, and wearing flats the rest of the time. I also spend lots of thinking of and adjusting my body position, walking and paying attention to my gait, and doing corrective exercises on a daily basis.

You can develop the movement program and footwear closet that suit you best, using *the way you feel* as a marker for any adjustments. Health is just like an outfit; you can style it however you'd like, so long as it makes you feel good.

ALIGNMENT, THE BIGGER PICTURE

You have learned about your feet and the importance of keeping them aligned for the sake of optimal physiological function, and minimal degeneration. Even though this concept is applied to the topic of foot pain, the theory applies equally across the entire body.

There are many ailments that stem from the lack of movement that comes from limitations (i.e., casts) we have placed on our bodies, like shoes, chairs, and cars, to name a few. To some, alignment solutions seem too simple to actually work. "If changing how I moved really worked, wouldn't I have been given that information already?" The reality is, many people would prefer a simple fix, and so the solutions have gone by way of a pill you can ingest in a moment, or a surgery that requires six weeks of your life. Corrective exercise isn't sexy and it isn't fast. But it does, in most cases, address the problem and not the symptom. And that's why many people finally arrive at this type of solution when they have experienced a recurrence of their issue despite numerous treatments.

Don't get me wrong: I believe there is absolutely an appropriate place and time for complex treatments when they're warranted, but these should fall in line after eliminating the most basic, mechanical causes of tissue damage. To seek healing in the very same environment that created the injury is like trying to lose weight eating exactly the same diet that brought it on. Physiology works in a very particular way; this book is written to help you consider and work *with your body* to find the outcomes you desire.

Key Points, Chapter 9

1. You absolutely do not need to scrap all the shoes in your closet to improve your current state of foot health.

2. If you need to purchase a shoe that is aligned with healthy-shoe criteria (see chapter 5), pick a model that you will be wearing while logging most of your weekly walking miles.

3. Your rate of improvement is a function of how much time you spend breaking old habits and starting new, better habits of body use.

4. Your alignment matters to the health of your entire body.

5. Changing mechanical causes of ailments is a fairly simple, easy, and inexpensive way to work toward relief.

CHAPTER 10

Guidelines, Recommendations, and Frequently Asked Questions

The following pages are an integration of everything this book has covered, and how to use the information to make logical, healthy decisions when it comes to footwear and foot care. So let's start from the beginning—the very beginning . . .

A good timeline for foot health and development should begin in childhood, one would think. However, because so much of a child's development hinges on what the parent is doing, I like to start my recommendations with pregnancy, because it is never too early to start modeling good behavior. Also, reading through this timeline may help you figure out (if you haven't already) where your personal foot experience was affected along the way.

A BABY ON THE WAY

Let's talk for a moment about pregnancy. Let's talk about the extra weight, all loaded onto the midsection. The lack of flexibility, the difficulty putting on shoes, and the swollen ankles. I might also mention the back pain and pregnancy-induced sciatica, so very common these days. And I won't mention the nausea, so fresh in my mind (I wrote the first edition while emerging from my first trimester; I'm happy to say I can no longer remember that period of my pregnancy well).

All of these ailments, now a common part of pregnancy, actually are not a direct result of pregnancy, but a combination of extra weight loaded onto a frame that came to pregnancy with footwear-altered geometry. With geometrical changes happening left and right, front and back, this is the perfect time to develop habits that support your body well.

Because footwear affects joint position from the ankles all the way up to (and through) the spine, placing these malaligned body parts under a steadily increasing weight can make ailments of the foot (and lower leg) develop more quickly.

Other considerations specific to pregnancy are the potential changes to pelvic alignment that your footwear produces. When the pelvis is taken out of alignment, the mobility of the muscles in the hips and pelvic girdle can change, which, in turn, can affect the mechanics of delivery. Many women will work on muscle and joint mobility via various prenatal exercise classes, so consider what you're putting on your feet and make sure your footwear isn't inadvertently working against you and your birth plan.

For the sake of comfort, health, and better mechanics before and during delivery, stick (or transition) to flat shoes, and spend lots of time opening the muscles in the feet, lower legs, and backs of the thighs. An extra bonus to keeping your pelvis stacked over your hips (as opposed to wearing it out in front of you) during pregnancy is enjoying the extra support your skeleton can lend to the increasing mass, as opposed to letting certain muscles and ligaments bear the load.

KIDS

Childhood is a great time to start integrating all of the information in this book. The problem is that you're probably already grown up. And maybe you already have kids, or maybe your children already have children of their own. Either way, you can now offer lots of advice from this section to others on what footwear they should choose for their kids. Because everyone loves parenting advice. Am I right?

Before you start picking out the perfect footwear for your children I want to clearly state that there is no footwear required for correct foot development. Those of you who grew up in households where footwear was mandatory—"Make sure you have your shoes on before you go outside!"—will be surprised. Yes, the human foot develops quite nicely, and likely even better, without shoes. I say this despite my own painful memory of having a fish hook taken out of my foot in the middle of a camping trip, and a less painful memory (for me) of my sister stepping onto a nail sticking out of a board (she was about ten years old, on the phone with a boy, and no, she didn't even drop the phone). While the human foot does not require shoes, the reality is, the barefoot time required for natural foot development isn't always the safest option when we're surrounded with manmade surfaces and detritus.

The best solution I have is to look for special children's brands that offer extreme flexibility, as well as lots of space to spread their toes. Keep in mind that children grow extremely fast, meaning that a shoe that fits today is swiftly on its way to becoming too small tomorrow, which can get expensive for sure. I've worked with many adults who recall squishing into hand-me-downs, having to curl toes to prevent them from banging into their shoes near the end of the school year, and going barefoot in the summer before next year's shoes came in the fall. Buying shoes for the kids still tends to be dictated by the season rather than by the needs of the foot, but remember: the foot needs space to move and grow.

Babies really require lots of barefoot time, especially when learning to crawl and walk. Beyond temperature control in extreme climates, socks can also limit motor development. As infants learn to move, a sock against a tile or hard wood floor inhibits development of the essential "push off" part of human gait. If you've ever spent any time on ice or snow, trying to walk without falling, your resultant movement pattern is not your best way of walking: it's only how you cope with this particular terrain. When you couple socks with a slick surface (both fairly unnatural occurrences in nature) you get something similar to ice walking. Slick surfaces can interfere with the natural gait development process because you've introduced forces that aren't there naturally. Your muscle patterns can stay with you for life, so pay attention to your babies when they're on the move and look for socks or surfaces that offer traction. It is definitely worth it in the long run of natural movement development.

And, speaking of kids, here's something to consider: the body establishes the level of maximum ("peak") bone mineral density around age twenty. The upright, weight-bearing motions that develop bone happen abundantly in kids— they've got a lot of energy and natural tendency to stay active. Putting a heel under their feet during this critical phase of bone development can penalize them for the rest of their life simply because of the geometry created at the ankle. Sadly, you can't develop your bone reserves beyond the amount established during this development phase. My suggestion is to forgo the trendy mini-fashions for long-term skeletal longevity, and your kids can choose once they're older.

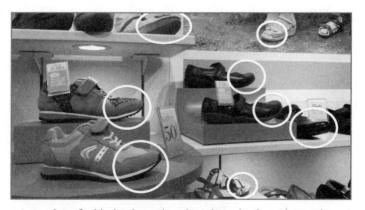

It's tough to find kids' shoes that don't have heels and raised toes!
(Photo credit: Ariana Rabinovitch)

SHOES AT THE OFFICE

I do a lot of magazine interviews and reporters are always asking me for tips "for the woman who *has* to wear high heels." I am always happy to offer tips, but I want to know: Who exactly is requiring women to wear heels? Seriously, if you've got "wearing heels" listed on your job contract, this might warrant a discussion with the Occupational Safety and Health Administration.

That being said, if you wear heels because you feel they make you seem more professional, then you are going to have to do the exercises in this book on a more regular basis. The exercises are designed to help you lengthen and strengthen all of the tissues most commonly shortened and weakened by certain parts of footwear. Keep in mind that the time you spend in shoes with geometry-altering components is time spent shortening all your tissues you've just worked to lengthen.

If you are wearing positive-heeled shoes all the time—meaning not only are your work and casual shoes elevated above a flat but your athletic shoes have at least an inch under the back, you will find it takes a lot longer to get out a foot crisis.

Here are some tips to quicken the pace:

- Get a pair of flat walking shoes to ensure that your fitness-walking time improves not only your fitness level but also the function of your feet.
- Keep a pair of flats in your desk at work. When you find yourself needing to walk for an errand

in the office, or if your feet end up feeling particularly limited in that day's shoes, slip on your backups. I have found that a pair of neutral, all-leather flats is suitable for most every outfit.

- Take a few 3- to 5-minute breaks within the workday to do your exercises.
- Get a pair of toe-alignment socks or toe spacers to slip on when you get home from work. This will give you a lot more time in the "spread out" toe position than just running through the exercises now and then.

SENIORS

Footwear research has tended to focus often on older adults. The reason? Foot pain has been associated with lack of mobility, balance, and self-efficacy in this population, and researchers want to know what can be done to improve the situation. One of the interesting findings in these studies is the prevalence of poor footwear fit, in both men and women. As tissues deform under years of loading (and misloading), the feet change in shape and size. The problem? Many seniors tend to wear the same shoes, or purchase new shoes without having their feet measured to see how their feet have changed.

It is often recommended that seniors begin purchasing shoes that offer large amounts of stability, meaning limited flexibility in the sole—very flat, very sturdy, etc. This suggestion is suitable for seniors who are not actively seeking to improve the health of their muscular system with regular exercise, balance therapy, or specific-movement classes. There is a fine line between creating a stable environment to avoid injury, and impeding muscle development with the same measure.

A happy medium, I think, is to create a safe space for exercising barefoot and doing balance-improving exercises, and otherwise using two main types of shoe. One should be less rigid for mindful sessions of gait improvement, and the other pair more structured when you're needing to go fast and not paying as much attention to where you're walking.

BONUS: A SIMPLE EXERCISE TO IMPROVE BALANCE

Stand in unshod feet, holding lightly to the back of a chair for support. Align the hips so they stack directly above the ankles. Make sure you can lift and wiggle the toes, demonstrating that your weight is far enough back over your heels.

Keeping both legs straight (it's very important that you don't bend either knee), push the right leg down into the floor, and let your left hip lift up away from the floor. Again (because I know how your knees want to cheat!), avoid bending the knees.

Keep your arms and shoulders relaxed and pay attention to how still (or not) your foot and ankle are. Practice this on a regular basis until you notice you are able to balance better and stay calm (relaxed shoulders, neck, face, etc.) while standing on one leg.

This is a simple exercise, but frankly, people don't actually realize how their stiff feet are contributing to their instability until they test their balance!

ALL NATURAL, ALL OF THE TIME

The "barefoot movement," new at the time of this book's first edition, has really taken off in the last few years due to some good books and magazine articles, and lots and lots of foot pain. Shoes were always assumed to be the best for foot health, and through investigation it has turned out that there's likely a balance between wearing shoes (in situations with great risk) and being barefoot (all of the other time) that's best for the body.

I really love the barefoot movement, but what I would have really, *really* loved would have been the barefoot movement starting about a hundred years ago, before it seemed like a good idea to lay down concrete and asphalt everywhere. That all of our foot parts need to move for the entire foot to function well is self-evident. Similarly, it should be self-evident that this doesn't just mean "no shoes" but also natural surfaces—those that give and also vary in shape, slope, and texture.

We need to train smart and be logical. If you want natural foot movements for optimal health, walk in natural environments. Shoes have been protecting us from our over-rigid environment for some time, and it takes time (years, even) to restore function. To get those feet healthier quicker, I strongly suggest a plan for increasing range of motion and function of the intrinsic foot musculature, and restoring appropriate length to extrinsic foot, lower leg, and thigh muscles.

I regularly see people get excited over the latest training fad, and then running out and buying the new barefoot-simulating shoes so they can run in a way that is "better for their health." I see these same people take feet that have no motor skill or strength, slap on their new shoes, and take a long run on paved streets in their neighborhood, their upper body falling out in front of them, increasing the g-forces of their landing with every step. Slap! Slap! Slap!

You want to go *au naturel*? Here are some guidelines to slowly transition yourself from a shoe-wearer to a minimalist.

1. Start with a daily stretching and massage of the heels, midfoot, forefoot, and toes.
2. Do your foot exercises—a lot. No, really, I mean it. Do them *all the time*.
3. Understand that the position of the foot is maintained by the muscles of the hips and make sure you optimize lateral hip (iliotibial or "IT" band), hamstring, gluteal, and adductor (inner thigh) strength with stretching and full ranges of motion. Tight hips can limit foot mobility and function.
4. Get a super-flexible shoe with a minimal (or better yet, no) heel.
5. Before jumping into non-shoe shoes, deal with your whole-body alignment and gait mechanics.

Podiatrists are seeing a huge increase in forefoot fractures from people (even highly experienced runners) who land with excessive force on the front of the foot. Walking should be heel to toe, not landing on the front of the foot. Running should be done on natural surfaces with body weight stacked correctly (without the torso leaning forward).

6. If you get non-shoe shoes, be a walker. If you do choose to run, build up your walking mileage for at least a year before even considering running in them.

7. Log your miles on a natural surface, with elevation changes and rocky obstacles. The urban jungle is not a natural walking surface; the hardness and traction of this surface can be an unnatural match to the human body.

An interesting note: Barefoot parks, or outdoor areas that are dedicated to offering debris-free trails, pebbly surfaces, and plenty of in-nature, balance-challenging obstacles are beginning to pop up as more people become aware of our waning foot strength. Currently these parks are available mostly in Europe, but hopefully in time, their importance will be recognized and developed in schools and public parks throughout the entire shoe-wearing world.

FAQs

There are a few questions that I am asked repeatedly regarding feet, footwear, and special considerations. Hopefully your question is found somewhere on these pages!

Is there ever a right time for . . . ?

Flip-Flops

Sure. As basic foot protection in a public bathing area, for getting in and out of the pool, or for walking on the beach, these bikini-esque shoes are fine. The negative impact of this type of footwear only comes from wearing it often, creating certain muscular recruitment.

If you like the open feel of a flip-flop, try to find a shoe with a minimal yet well-engineered upper that gives you plenty of breathing room across the feet without invoking alterations in your stride or your foot-firing patterns. There are many outdoor-shoe companies that strive to offer in- and out-of-the-water footwear that make water sports and outdoor activities safe for the feet, yet a lot more comfortable than a full, heavy shoe.

High Heels

I am sure by this point you think I hate fashion, but that's not true at all. I love cute shoes just as much as the next person. I just happen to love geometry a whole lot more. High-heeled shoes are fine to wear on those special occasions. Again, it is just the enduring habit of wearing these shoes that racks up the long-term damage. If you do happen to take the shoes out for a night on the town, you are more than likely going to have a High Heel Hangover to deal with the next day.

For feet not used to wearing killers, the hangover can be blisters, burning in the front of the foot, sore toes, tender lower legs, calf cramps, or next-day back pain. Give yourself time to do a few gentle passes over the exercises. To really loosen everything up, give yourself 5 minutes of foot exercise for every hour you spent in your shoes. When done, the skin of the feet may still be sensitive, but the muscles should feel a whole lot better.

P.S. If you happen to sprain your ankle while wearing these shoes, it is best not to tell me. I'll only say, "I told you so," and then tell you to do your exercises once it heals.

What about orthotics?

When foot tissues fail to maintain their structural integrity, it can allow structures to displace—the ankles, for example. Because the ankles are at the bottom of a long chain of other joints, moving them can create a chain reaction that affects the knees and hips.

Movement of the hips can affect the musculature of the pelvic floor, the abdominals, and the spine, as many of these muscles attach to the bones in the legs.

As you can tell from this book, if the feet aren't doing their job, it is really important to rectify the situation. Orthotics is one way to prevent the entire structure from collapsing. However, the orthotic is not a foot-strengthening apparatus. The orthotic is essentially a support for the bones in lieu of the muscles doing their job.

Because you've read this deeply into the book, you will probably realize that I am about to tell you that in addition to using your orthotics, you might consider undertaking a foot-strengthening program.

I've been wearing heels for a long time. Is it safe to drop down into flats?

If you've been wearing a high, positive-heeled shoe for a long time, it will take some time before your tissue releases enough to allow you to wear lower shoes comfortably and safely. Before changing footwear, start with this book's foot exercise program to gradually prepare your tissues. Stretching the calves is a real eye-opener for most people. If you can barely stretch your calves using the stretch from this book, you can wait a while before changing shoes.

That said, find the lowest heel height you feel physically comfortable in and set that as your new "highest" heel. You can start working your way down from this new height, making progress that is accordant to the time you spend retraining your foot muscles and paying attention to your gait pattern.

Why is my doctor prescribing heels for my plantar fasciitis?

This is an old, easy "solution" to the pain that develops with extreme tension in the lower leg, Achilles' tendon, or heel of the foot. The rationale is, your tissues are so tight that simply dropping your heel down to the floor during the regular gait cycle is enough to tear the tissue, so keep the heels from touching (i.e., wear shoes that prevent your heel from getting to the ground).

If you continue with a tension-making gait pattern that incorrectly loads foot and lower-leg tissues, the problem continues to worsen until you are right back where you started—suffering the pain of plantar fasciitis.

What to do? If you are currently unable to walk without a heel, see the earlier recommendation for those who have been wearing heels for a long time. The secret to dealing successfully with this issue is diligence—both in doing the exercises regularly, and in paying attention to how you carry your body over your foot while walking and standing.

What if I want to wear shoes that are good for my feet most of the time, but still keep some of my old habits? Will that make any difference at all?

Keep in mind that the changes brought about by a positive heel are similar to the physiological changes brought about by a really delicious dessert, like crème brûlée. Just because you eat crème brûlée every now and then doesn't mean that you've abandoned eating well most of the time. The same goes for footwear. When you splurge, it is just that—a splurge. Come home and work it out in the foot gym. A pair of flat or negative-heeled shoes are doing good whenever they are on your feet and nothing can take that away from you, not even a stroll down the shoe-candy aisle every now and then!

Key Points, Chapter 10

1. Footwear should always be selected thoughtfully, as shoes can impact structures beyond the feet.
2. Selecting appropriate footwear for children is important, as this is the time when they are developing habits and tissues that will last them a lifetime.
3. There is a right time and right place for all footwear, but there is also a corresponding need to deal with after-effects using exercise and other suggestions.
4. Because each of us has a unique "user's pattern" in our feet, the exercise program should be modified based on where you are right now, with a change in footwear happening gradually—especially in those with deeply engrained foot-tension patterns.

EXERCISES AND POSITIONS TO KEEP HEALTHY FEET

FEET STRAIGHT

- Line up the OUTSIDE EDGE of each foot with a straight edge, like a plank in a wood floor (don't worry if some parts of your foot fall over the line).
- If this points your toes inward, don't worry; they will adjust their position with time and practice of the other exercises.

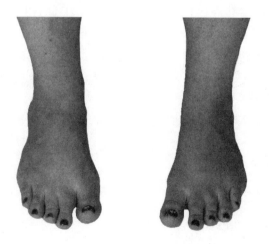

ANKLE TO HIP ON A VERTICAL LINE

- Standing sideways to a
  mirror, hold a yardstick
  perpendicular to the
  ground (showing a vertical
  line).
- Still sideways, position your
  ankle to the bottom of the
  stick, and bring the center
  of your pelvis onto the line.
- Keep your knees straight,
  but kneecaps down.

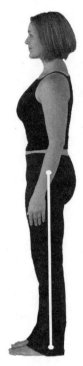

MOVE THE TOES INDIVIDUALLY

- Start by raising the big
  toe without moving any
  of the others.
- Then raise the second,
  third, fourth, and fifth,
  one at a time.
- Like you can move your
  fingers, practice moving
  your toes individually (or
  practice trying!).

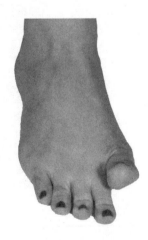

STRETCH THE CALVES

- Feet pointed straight ahead.
- Heel on the ground.
- Hips stay vertical over back ankle.

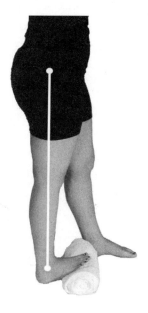

STRETCH YOUR TOES

- Grab your left foot with your right hand, and vice versa.
- For more stretch, lace your fingers deeper between the toes, closer to the foot.

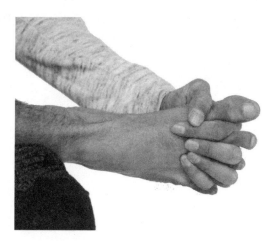

FOOT ON BALL

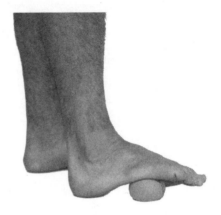

- Stand (or sit for less pressure) with your feet side by side.
- Keep your heel on the ground and press your forefoot onto a tennis ball.
- Move the ball to different parts of the sole, applying continuous pressure. Hold each location for 20 to 30 seconds.

FORWARD FOLD AGAINST A WALL

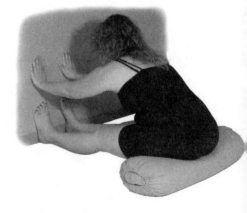

- Sit on a rolled towel or cushion, keeping the knees and thighs relaxed and straight.
- Press your heels into the wall.
- Reach your hands to the wall, folding at the level of the hips instead of along the spine.
- Take relaxing breaths, and do not bounce.

LENGTHEN THE BACKS OF THE LEGS

- Stand facing a chair with legs straight at the knees.
- Keep the feet straight, heels on the ground, forefeet raised onto a towel.
- Fold forward from the hips (not the spine) and let the tip of your tailbone rise up and away from the ground.

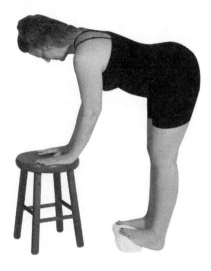

STRETCHING THE GRIPPING MUSCLES

- Starting with the toenails, lay down the top of the foot behind you, keeping the heel centered.
- For more stretch, straighten the back knee and reach back from the hip.

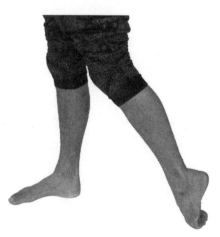

SPREAD YOUR TOES

- Stand or sit with your feet pointed straight ahead.
- Practice spreading your toes away from each other—side to side, but not up or down.

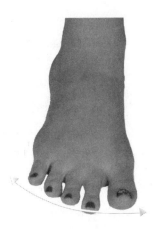

APPENDIX

I maintain several lists of minimalist shoes on my website, where you can find:

- general recommendations in my Shoes: The List post (nutritiousmovement.com/shoes-the-list)
- warm-weather recommendations in my Shoes: The Summer List post (nutritiousmovement.com /shoes-the-summer-list)
- cold-weather recommendations in my Shoes: The Winter List post (nutritiousmovement.com /shoes-the-winter-list).

Toe Spacers

MY-HAPPY FEET ORIGINAL ALIGNMENT SOCK
www.my-happyfeet.com

CORRECT TOES
https://nwfootankle.com/correct-toes

Cobblestone Walking Mats

www.allegromedical.com

www.gaiam.com

Self-Massage Therapy Balls

Yogatuneup.com

REFERENCES AND
ADDITIONAL READING

Arnadottir, S., and V. Mercer. 2000. Effects of footwear on measurements of balance and gait in women between the ages of 65 and 93 years. *Physical Therapy* 80 (1): 17-27.

Barnett, C. 1962. The normal orientation of the human hallux and the effect of footwear. *Journal of Anatomy* 96 (Part 4): 489-94.1.

Barnicot, N.A. 1955. The position of the hallux in West Africans. *Journal of Anatomy* 89 (Part 3): 355–61.

Bendix, T., S. Sorensen, and K. Klausen. 1984. Lumbar curve, trunk muscles, and line of gravity with different heel heights. *Spine* 9 (2): 223-27.

Bergmann, G., H. Kniggendorf, F. Graichen, and A. Rohlmann. 1995. Influence of shoes and heel strike on the loading of the hip joint. *Journal of Biomechanics* 28 (7): 817-27.

Birn-Jeffery, A.V., and T.E. Higham. 2014. The scaling of uphill and downhill locomotion in legged animals. *Integrative and Comparative Biology*. [Epub ahead of print]

Carl, T., S. Barrett. 2008. Computerized analysis of plantar pressure variation in flip-flops, athletic shoes, and bare feet. *Journal of the American Podiatric Medical Association* 98 (5): 374-78.

Carpenter, K.J. 2012. The discovery of vitamin C. *Annals of Nutrition and Metabolism* 61(3): 259-64.

Chevalier, Gaétan, S. T. Sinatra, J. L. Oschman, K. Sokal, and P. Sokal. 2012. Earthing: health implications of reconnecting the human body to the Earth's surface electrons. *Journal of Environmental and Public Health*, Article ID 291541: 1-8.

Cho, N.H., S. Kim, D.J. Kwon, and H.A. Kim. 2009. The prevalence of hallux valgus and its association with foot pain and function in a rural Korean community. *Journal of Bone and Joint Surgery*—British Volume 91 (4): 494-98.

Crockett, H., B. Gross, K. Wilk, M. Schwartz, J. Reed, J. O'Mara & J. Andrews. 2000. Osseous adaptation and range of motion at the gleno-humeral joint in professional baseball. *The American Journal of Sports Medicine* 30 (1): 20-26.

Csapo, R., C. Maganaris, O. Seynnes, and M. Narici. 2010. On muscle, tendon and high heels. *Journal of Experimental Biology* 213: 2582-88.

Daoût, K., T. Pataky, D. De Clercq, and P. Aerts. 2009. The effects of habitual footwear use: foot shape and function in native barefoot walkers. *Footwear Science* 1 (2): 81-94.

Dawson, J., M. Thorogood, S. Marks, E. Juszczak, C. Dodd, G. Lavis, and R. Fitzpatrick. 2002. The prevalence of foot problems in older women: a cause for concern. *Journal of Public Health* 24 (2): 77-84.

de Lateur, B., R. Giaconi, K. Questad, M. Ko, and J. Lehmann. 1991. Footwear and posture: compensatory strategies for heel height. *American Journal of Physical Medicine Rehabilitation* 70 (5): 246-54.

De Wit, B., D. De Clercq, and P. Aerts. 2000. Biomechanical analysis of the stance phase during barefoot and shod running. *Journal of Biomechanics* 33 (3): 269-78.

Eisenhardt, J., D. Cook, I. Pregler, and H. Foehl. 1996. Changes in temporal gait characteristics and pressure distribution for bare feet versus various heel heights. *Gait and Posture* 4 (4): 280-86.

Esenyel, M., K. Walsh, J. Walden, A. Gitter. 2003. Kinetics of high-heeled gait. *Journal of the American Podiatric Medical Association* 93 (1): 27-32.

Fanchiang, Hsin-chen and Geil, Mark D. 2014. The effects of walking surface and vibration on the gait pattern and vibration perception threshold of typically developing children and children with idiopathic toe walking. Dissertation, Georgia State University.

Frey, C., F. Thompson, J. Smith, M. Sanders, and H. Horstman. 1993. American Orthopedic Foot and Ankle Society women's shoe survey. *Foot and Ankle* 14 (2): 78-81.

Fulkerson, J., E. Arendt, L. Griffin, J. Garrick. 2002. Anterior knee pain in females. *Clinical Orthopedics & Related Research* 372 (March): 69-73.

Gabell, A., M. Simons, U. Nayak. 1985. Falls in the healthy elderly: predisposing causes. *Ergonomics* 28 (7): 965-75.

Gefen, A., M. Megido-Ravid, Y. Itzchak, and M. Arcan. 2001. Analysis of muscular fatigue and foot stability during high-heeled gait. *Gait and Posture* 15 (1): 56-63.

Giuliani, Jeffrey; B. Masini, C. Alitz, B. D. Owens. 2011. Barefoot-simulating footwear associated with metatarsal stress injury in two runners. **Healio Orthopedics** 34 (7): e320-e323).

Gottschalk F., J. Sallis, P. Beighton, and L. Solomon. 1980. A comparison of the prevalence of hallux valgus in three South African populations. *South African Medical Journal* 57 (10): 355-57.

Hill, C., T. Gill, H. Menz, and A. Taylor. 2008. Prevalence and correlates of foot pain in a population-based study: the North West Adelaide health study. *Journal of Foot and Ankle Research*, July 28, 2008.

Jenkins, D. W. and D. J. Cauthon. 2011. Barefoot running claims and controversies. *Journal of the American Podiatric Medical Association* 101 (3): 231-246.

Kerrigan, D., J. Johansson, M. Bryant, J. Boxer, U. Croce, and P. Riley. 2005. Moderate-heeled shoes and knee joint torques relevant to the development and progression of knee osteoarthritis. *Physical Medicine and Rehabilitation* 86 (5): 871-75.

Kerrigan, D., J. Lelas, and M. Karvosky. 2001. Women's shoes and knee osteoarthritis. *The Lancet* 357 (9262): 1097-98.

Kerrigan, D., M. Todd, and P. Riley. 1998. Knee osteoarthritis and high-heeled shoes. *The Lancet* 351 (9113): 1399-1401.

Kirby, K. A. 2001. Subtalar joint axis location and rotational equilibrium theory of foot function. *Journal of the American Podiatric Medical Association* 91 (9): 465-487.

Lee, C., E. Jeong, and A. Freivalds. 2001. Biomechanical effects of wearing high-heeled shoes. *International Journal of Industrial Ergonomics* 28 (6): 321-26.

Lieberman, Daniel E., M. Venkadesan, W.A. Werbel, A. I. Daoud, S. D'Andrea, I.S. Davis, R. Ojiambo Mang'Eni & Y. Pitsiladis. *2010. Foot strike patterns and collision forces in habitually barefoot versus shod runners. Nature 463: 531-535.*

Maclennan, R. 1966. Prevalence of hallux valgus in a neolithic New Guinea population. *The Lancet* 287 (7452): 1398-1400.

Martin, R. Bruce, David Burr, & Neil A. Sharkey. 1998. *Skeletal Tissue Mechanics.* New York: Springer-Verlag.

McBride I., U. Wyss, T. Cooke, L. Murphy, J. Phillips, and S. Olney. 1991. First metatarsophalangeal joint reaction forces during high-heel gait. *Foot and Ankle* 11 (5): 282-88.

Menz, H.B., and M.E. Morris. 2005. Footwear characteristics and foot problems in older people. *Gerontology* 51 (5): 346-51.

Menz, H.B., A. Tiedemann, M.M. Kwan, K. Plumb, and S.R. Lord. 2007. Foot pain in community-dwelling older people: an evaluation of the Manchester Foot Pain and Disability Index. *Rheumatology* (Oxford) 46 (2): 375.

Menz, H.B., E. Roddy, E. Thomas, and P. Croft. 2011. Impact of hallux valgus severity on general and foot-specific health-related quality of life. *Arthritis Care and Research* 63 (6): 396-404.

Morgan, Christopher. 2008. Reconstructing pre-historic hunter-gatherer foraging radii: a case study from California's southern Sierra Nevada. *Journal of Archaeological Science* 35 (2): 247-258.

Mullaji A.B., A.K. Sharma, S.V. Marawar, A. F. Kohli. 2008. Tibial torsion in non-arthritic Indian adults: A computer tomography study of 100 limbs. *Indian Journal of Orthopaedics* 42 (3): 309-13.

Nigg, B. 2001. The role of impact forces and foot pronation: a new paradigm. *Clinical Journal of Sports Medicine* 11 (1): 2-9.

Nix, S., M. Smith, and B. Vicenzino. 2010. Prevalence of hallux valgus in the general population: a systematic review and meta-analysis. *Journal of Foot and Ankle Research* 3 (September 27): 21.

Nurse, M.A., et al. 2005. Changing the texture of footwear can alter gait patterns. *Journal of Electromyography and Kinesiology* 15 (5): 496-506.

Raichlen, D.A., B.M. Wood, A.D. Gordon, A.Z. Mabulla, F.W. Marlowe and H. Pontzer. 2014. Evidence of Levy walk foraging patterns in human hunter-gatherers. *Proceedings of the National Academy of Sciences* 111(2): 728-33.

Rao, U., and B. Joseph. 1992. The influence of footwear on the prevalence of flat foot. A survey of 2300 children. *The Journal of Bone and Joint Surgery* 74 (4): 525-27.

Ridge, Sarah T.; Johnson, A. Wayne; Mitchell, Ulrike H.; Hunter, Iain; Robinson, Eric; Rich, Brent S. E.; Brown, Stephen Douglas. 2013. Foot bone marrow edema after 10-week transition to minimalist running shoes. *Medicine & Science in Sports & Exercise* 45 (7): 1363-8.

Rixe, Jeffrey A., R.A. Gallo, M.L. Silvis. 2012. The barefoot debate: can minimalist shoes reduce running-related injuries? *Current Sports Medicine Report* 11 (3): 160-65.

Robbins, S., and A. Hanna. 1987. Running-related injury prevention through barefoot adaptations. *Medicine and Science in Sports and Exercise* 19 (2): 148-56.

Robbins, S., G. Gouw, and A. Hanna. 1989. Running-related injury prevention through innate impact-moderating behavior. *Medicine and Science in Sports and Exercise* 21 (2): 130-39.

Rome, K., D. Hancock, and D. Poratt. 2008. Barefoot running and walking: the pros and cons based on current evidence. *The New Zealand Medical Journal* 121 (1272).

Rossi, William A. 1999. Why shoes make 'normal' gait impossible. *Podiatry Management* (March): 50-61.

Rossi, W. 2001. Footwear: the primary cause of foot disorders. A continuation of the scientific review of the failings of modern shoes. *Podiatry Management* (February): 129-38.

Shaw, C.N. and Stock, J.T. 2009. Habitual throwing and swimming correspond with upper limb diaphyseal strength and shape in modern human athletes. *American Journal of Physical Anthropology* 140 (1): 160-172.

Sherrington, C., and H. Menz. 2002. An evaluation of footwear worn at the time of fall-related hip fracture. *Age and Aging* 32 (3): 310-14.

Shroyer, J., and W. Weimar. 2010. Comparative analysis of human gait while wearing thong-style flip-flops versus sneakers. *Journal of the American Podiatric Medical Association* 100 (4): 251-57.

Shull, P.B., R. Shultz, A. Slider, J.L. Dragoo, T.F. Besier and S. L. Delp. 2013. Toe-in gait reduces the first peak knee adduction moment in patients with medial compartment knee osteoarthritis. *Journal of Biomechanics*, 46 (1), 122-128.

Sládek, V., M. Berner, R. Sailer. 2006. Mobility in Central European Late Eneolithic and Early Bronze Age: Tibial Cross-sectional Geometry. *Journal of Archaeological Science* 33 (4): 470–482.

Venkataraman, V.V., T.S. Kraft, J.M. Desilva and N.J. Dominy. 2013. Phenotypic plasticity of climbing-related traits in the ankle joint of great apes and rainforest hunter-gatherers. *Human Biology,* 85(1-3): 309-28.

Venkataraman, V.V., T.S. Kraft and N.J. Dominy. 2013. Tree climbing and human evolution. *Proceedings of the National Academy of Sciences of the United States of America* 110 (4): 1237-42.

Villamin, C.A.C., and J.F.C. Syquia. 2012. Tibial torsion among Filipinos: a cavaderic study. *Malaysian Orthopedic Journal* 6 (3): 27-30.

von Tscharner, V., B. Goepfert, and B. Nigg. 2003. Changes in EMG signals for the muscle tibialis anterior while running barefoot or with shoes resolved by non-linearly scaled wavelets. *Journal of Biomechanics* 36 (8): 1169-76.

Vormittag, K., R. Calonje, and W.W. Briner. 2009. Foot and ankle injuries in the barefoot sport. *Current Sports Medicine Reports* 8 (5): 262-66.

Weist, Roger, E. Eils, D. Rosenbaum. 2004. The influence of muscle fatigue on electromyogram and plantar pressure patterns as an explanation for the incidence of metatarsal stress fractures. *American Journal of Sports Medicine* 32 (8): 1893-1898.

Willems, T., E. Witvrouw, A. De Cock, and D. De Clercq. 2007. Gait-related risk factors for exercise-related lower-leg pain during shod running. *Medicine and Science in Sports and Exercise* 39 (2): 330-39.

Zipfel, B. and L.R. Berger. 2007. Shod versus unshod: the emergence of forefoot pathology in modern humans. *The Foot* 17 (4): 205-13.

INDEX

ABOUT THE AUTHOR

A biomechanist by training and a problem-solver at heart, Katy has the ability to blend a scientific approach with straight talk about sensible solutions and an unwavering sense of humor, earning her legions of followers. Her award-winning blog and podcast, Katy Says, reach hundreds of thousands of people every month, and thousands have taken her live classes. Her books, the bestselling *Move Your DNA* (2014), *Diastasis Recti* (2016), *Whole Body Barefoot* (2015), *Alignment Matters* (2013), and *Every Woman's Guide to Foot Pain Relief* (2011), have been critically acclaimed and translated worldwide. In between her book-writing efforts, Katy directs and teaches at the Nutritious Movement Center Northwest in Washington state, travels the globe to teach the Nutritious Movement™ courses in person, and spends as much time outside as possible with her husband and two young children.